STRESS CONTROL THROUGH SELF-HYPNOSIS

❖ This book is dedicated to all
my patients who, throughout the years,
have taught me so much.

STRESS CONTROL THROUGH SELF-HYPNOSIS

DR ARTHUR JACKSON

Illustrations by Brian Kogler

PIATKUS

ACKNOWLEDGEMENTS

Producing a book such as this is a cooperative enterprise and many people contributed to its development. Although the initial concept was mine, the idea may well have lain fallow without the stimulation provided by Hazel Young, and Rex Finch and Ian Morton of Transworld Publishers. I am grateful to them for their continuing belief in my ability to produce this work.

I am deeply indebted to Rosemary Wildie who had to shoulder the huge burden of typing and retyping the manuscript. Rosemary confronted the formidable task of sifting through the vast amounts of copy with unfailing patience, accuracy and good humour and her efforts are greatly appreciated.

It was not possible for me to write this book without my becoming something of a social hermit and I owe a special debt of gratitude to my wife, Ann, for her wonderful support and understanding throughout. She also had the unenviable task of acting as a sounding board for my ideas, and provided so many helpful suggestions.

Finally, my thanks to Julie Stanton and Gill Hewitt for the invaluable editorial comments which helped shape the final result.

Text copyright © Dr Arthur Jackson
Illustrations © Brian Kogler

First published in Great Britain in 1990 by
Judy Piatkus (Publishers) Limited of
5 Windmill Street, London W1P 1HF

First paperback edition 1993

Published by arrangement
with Transworld Publishers
(Australia) Pty Ltd

A catalogue record for this book is available from
the British Library
ISBN 0–86188–959–2
0–7499–1209–X (pbk)

Cover design by Jennie Smith

Printed and bound in Great Britain by
Butler & Tanner Ltd, Frome and London

❖ CONTENTS ❖

FOREWORD

I first met Arthur Jackson socially at a barbecue at his Sydney home in 1974. We shared a lot of interests, principally cricket and classical music, and became firm friends.

It was not until 1977 however, that I benefitted from his hypnotherapy. The England team had finished a long and arduous tour of India and Sri Lanka, culminating in the Centenary Test match in Melbourne. Exhausted both physically and mentally, I arrived at Arthur's home for a few days' break before returning to the UK. Unable to wind down, Arthur suggested a session of hypnosis to relax me, and thinking I had nothing to lose, I accepted.

After the session I was transformed – totally relaxed. I was converted to hypnotherapy immediately.

Tony Greig, the England captain of the day, had made some constructive criticisms of my approach to the game and with Arthur's help I started remedying these faults through two courses of action. The first was to get much fitter through a programme of long distance running. The second was a series of hypnotherapy sessions to improve my mental approach. Arthur made me a cassette of his own voice so that I could learn to hypnotise myself at home.

I used to come home from cricket, physically exhausted and with a head still buzzing, literally, from the events of the day. A spell of self-hypnosis was like inserting a corkscrew into one's mind and unscrewing all the tension, leaving one completely relaxed and at peace with the world.

I am convinced that I would not have achieved the same success in cricket had I not learned the skills of self-hypnosis.

Bob Willis
October 1989

INTRODUCTION

It is Saturday morning and I am standing on the first tee at my golf club, contemplating how I am going to master the vagaries of the course. Nearby, fellow golfers are immersed in discussing their current cholesterol levels and the various dietary and other approaches they are pursuing in order to maintain their cholesterol readings within acceptable norms. Strange behaviour you think? Not really because it is a sign of the times, an indication that we are starting to become aware of how important it is for each of us to take a role in our health. Instead of waiting for disease to overtake us, we are, at last, realising that we can all play an active part in protecting ourselves from illness.

One of the most significant things that has happened on the health front in more recent times is the realisation that stress can have very damaging effects on the body as well as the mind. In the early days of my medical career, it was a rare event, indeed, to read any scientific papers relating to stress but all this has changed and more and more prestigious journals are publishing articles devoted to the subject.

If stress is so harmful, can we do anything to control it in ourselves? The unequivocal answer is *yes*, and this has provided the stimulation for this book. Stress can arise from many sources, such as exposure to severe cold or partaking in excessive exercise. But the type of stress I am referring to throughout arises from mental or emotional sources. This is by far the most common and constant type experienced by all of us. It is an everyday experience and although we tend to think it only happens in response to some major traumatic events in our life, this is not usually the case. More frequently it develops as the result of constant daily hassles—ones that tax our coping resources to the limit.

The aim of this book, in a nutshell, is to help you develop your own coping mechanisms so that you can deal with life events without becoming fazed by them. This may not be as simple a task as it first appears and requires a certain amount of diligence on your part. But the rewards justify the effort.

The techniques of self-hypnosis are readily learnt but I would have to admit that they are not as easy as resorting to the pill bottle. On the other hand, taking tranquillisers does little to improve your coping skills and, surely, this is the crux of the matter. If you wish to master stress, the answer lies in learning techniques that help you relax in *all* situations in life.

I make no apologies for not dealing with all aspects of illness that are caused by stress. Instead, I have selected those health problems which most commonly confront people. Rest assured, however, that if you are interested in developing a healthy lifestyle, self-hypnosis will help you achieve this goal. There could be no better way of expressing the aims of self-hypnosis than by echoing the thoughts of the Roman poet Juvenal who in 130 A.D. wrote:

'*Orandum est ut sit mens sana in corpore sano.*
Your prayer must be that you may have a sound mind in a sound body.'

Dr Arthur Jackson

CHAPTER ONE

STRESS AND HOW IT AFFECTS YOU

Stress has often been described as a disorder of the twentieth century, but this is not really an accurate statement. Throughout his existence man has been subjected to stress in one form or another. Ancient man would certainly have experienced stress arising from difficulties in finding food or being pursued by predators. The reason why we view it as a modern phenomenon is that we are now much more aware of the harmful effects that it can have on our health.

The role of the unconscious mind

The concept of stress might be easier to understand if you view your mind as being divided into two parts: the conscious and unconscious (what some people call the subconscious). The part of the mind that we are particularly interested in is the unconscious, although it is not possible to disregard conscious actions in our everyday life for these often have considerable influence on unconscious behaviours. For the sake of simplicity it is useful to view the unconscious mind as a sort of storage or filing system. In computer terms, you would call it the data bank of the brain.

1

The effects of life experiences

Throughout your life, you are subjected to a wide variety of experiences and these you absorb, storing them in your unconscious as part of the process of learning. Some experiences will be good, some bad, but all tend to be stored away to influence you later. They may lead to your developing certain behaviours which, in turn, become fixed as everyday responses. You develop certain skills or ways of dealing with life situations as the result of the information you acquire and store in your unconscious. Even if you are not aware of it happening, each day and each event that you experience becomes a learning process in some way or other.

What is stress?

Although we all know intuitively what is meant by stress, curiously it defies precise definition. Much of the controversy surrounding the term 'stress' has arisen because it has been interpreted in a variety of ways by writers. Some see it as the stimulus or factor which disturbs health (for example, 'That person/thing stresses me a great deal'). Others consider it to be the ill health which a person experiences as the result of something that has happened in their life (for example, 'I felt very stressed by what happened in my job and I'm sure that contributed to my heart attack'). Rather than get caught up in this semantic confusion, I like to think of stress as an interaction between events which can produce adverse effects on health (we call these stressors), and the way the body reacts to these stressors.

The good stress of life

Is all stress harmful to you? Not necessarily. A noted authority on stress, Dr Hans Selye, proposed that stress can be good and bad. The good stimulates us to cope with difficulties that arise in our lives; the bad leads to ill health. He regarded good stress (he termed it 'eustress')as any change in our environment that teaches us to cope, in a better manner, with things in our life. As an example of this type of stress you could cite a businessperson who has won a large business contract, or an architect who has the satisfaction of seeing a complex design taking shape. In each case the job demands may have been excessive but because the final outcome was satisfying, they proved stimulating rather than overwhelming to the individual. On the other hand, bad stress (Selye calls this 'distress') is the type of stress that tends to tax us beyond our limits. For many people, life is a constant battle to maintain a balance between eustress and distress.

Damaging stress

If stress in your life is continual it will result in your mind being subjected to an overload of stimuli. Each of us has a particular coping threshold and if this is exceeded, stress will result. If the mind was a simple electrical circuit, a stress overload would probably lead to the burning-out of a fuse. Because of the human brain's complexity, however, it does not do this, but, instead, tries to find ways of dealing with the situation. To add to the burden, and hence aggravate the situation still further, your thinking patterns become negative and lead to all sorts of self-doubts, loss of self-esteem and self-confidence. And so the vicious circle depicted below is set up:

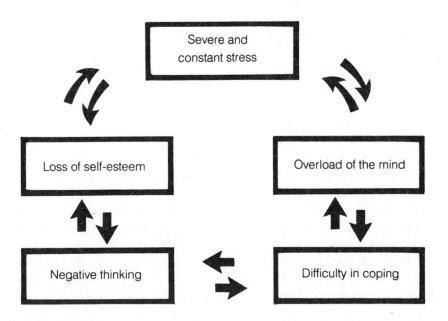

Once your mind becomes so overloaded with stress that it just cannot cope satisfactorily, it will indicate its distress by creating symptoms. These sometimes take on a physical form in the way of headaches, bowel disorders, pain, or skin problems; or they may be of a more psychological nature such as loss of confidence, loss of interest in work and home events, poor concentration and memory, or difficulty in sleeping. In such a situation, *everything* seems too much effort.

Why you become stressed

People's responses to a given set of conditions will differ widely. One person may, for example, handle a certain job situation with comparative ease whilst another will become distressed by the same work load. Why does this happen? There are many reasons why we behave differently. Some people are more inclined towards becoming easily stressed because they have inherited the tendency from their parents or forefathers. Such people could be described as stress-prone. But even if you do have this genetic predisposition to stress it does not necessarily mean that you are always going to suffer from it. You can build up your coping mechanisms through relaxation and by learning how to restructure your thoughts.

External factors can also influence the way you respond to daily pressures. These are things which lie much more under your control. We all recognise, for example, that we should take regular holidays, but in spite of this, not everyone does. This can be a very significant cause of stress. The work scene also often contributes in a major way to a person becoming stressed. It is not uncommon, especially in the business and professional worlds, for a person to be promoted to a position which lies beyond his or her capabilities. This phenomenon, known as the Peter Principle, was first humorously described by an American educator called Laurence Peter. Unfortunately, the increased demands and responsibility of being in a senior position can often prove excessive for someone who is ill-equipped to deal with them.

Lack of exercise, too, can play its part. It is widely recognised that regular exercise, in whatever form, helps to prevent you becoming stressed. One theory that has been advanced to account for this is that prolonged exercise causes the body to release into the bloodstream certain chemicals called endorphins. These are tranquilliser-like substances which lead to the feelings of well-being that joggers report after they have finished jogging.[1] The release of B-endorphin would explain why people who exercise regularly find that it acts as a de-stressor for them.

How can stress affect you?

Life is full of potential stressors; work, finance and family commitments can make you feel as though you are living in a pressure cooker.

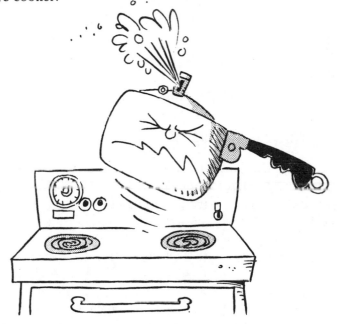

Life's stresses can give you a pressure cooker feeling

It is little wonder, therefore, that people are becoming more aware of stress as an important factor influencing their health and happiness. A recent study carried out at the Medicheck Centre in Sydney, Australia, showed that 42 per cent of women and 26 per cent of men considered themselves to be suffering from stress.[2] These figures, although significant, probably do not represent a true picture of its frequency in the population, for they only indicate when stress has actually been recognised as such by the patient. Many people find it difficult to acknowledge that their physical or mental symptoms are stress-related, especially when these problems have been evident for some time. They are more inclined to seek a physical explanation for their symptoms, a good example being people who suffer from headaches. These may be so severe and frequent that the person is convinced that something sinister, such as a brain tumour, is causing them. Although most headaches arise from tension and stress, it may be necessary for the person's doctor to carry out detailed investigations to exclude the presence of, say, a tumour. Once reassured, the person is likely then to agree to treatment of the *true* cause of their headaches—the stress and tension.

Stress can affect you both physically and mentally. Although both aspects are usually evident, by and large most of us tend to be much more aware of the symptoms created in the body than those arising in the mind.

Children and stress

We tend to think of stress as being solely an adult concern, but this is not true. Children, in fact, are most susceptible to becoming stressed. Their nervous systems are not fully developed and they have not yet had the opportunity to develop adequate coping skills.

When stress occurs in a child it usually presents differently from the way it does in an adult. Whereas a grown-up can recognise and freely admit to feeling tense, 'uptight', or finding it difficult to cope, a child does not have this ability. For this reason, children will often manifest their stress in a variety of behavioural ways. They may become disobedient at home, show a resentment of authority, and become generally untidy in their appearance. At school, academic standards may decline and the child may have difficulty keeping pace with class peers. At the outer end of the scale, stress can express itself through stealing, drug-taking or clashes with authority. Sometimes mental tension leads to physical problems such as asthma or bedwetting. Probably the most damaging effect of stress in any child is the way it lowers self-esteem. The young person loses all self-belief and this can soon interfere, for example, with how he or she relates to other children or the completion of school assignments.

Behavioural changes indicate that the child is stressed. In a sense they are a cry for help. If they are not recognised as such by parents, the child's behaviour will tend to worsen. This usually results in the parents becoming even more frustrated and hostile towards their offspring, serving to further intensify the stress factor.

Ways of helping the stressed child are outlined in Chapter 8.

STRESS AND YOUR BODY

The effects of muscle tension

The most common effects of stress are felt in the voluntary muscles and are experienced as muscle tension. Muscle tension can occur in any part of the body, but some muscle groups seem more prone to tension than others. The most common sites are the neck, the muscles of the face, the back of the head, between the shoulder blades, the lower back and the limbs. Sometimes this tension is felt as a constant tightness in the muscles—what some people describe as a 'knotted-up' sensation. This is a very apt description because, in fact, the muscle fibres of the affected region *are* in spasm. Such spasms will cause pain and tightness and sometimes there will be difficulty in moving that part of the body.

Contrary to what many people believe, this body tension is often not restricted to the waking hours. It is not uncommon for people who are tense to wake up each morning with facial pain because they have been clenching or grinding their teeth, or with their forearm muscles aching because they have been clinging tightly to the bedclothes in their sleep. This may strike you as strange, for don't we relax when we are asleep? The simple answer is no. It is important to realise that when you are stressed or anxious, this state will affect you in some way or other twenty-four hours a day.

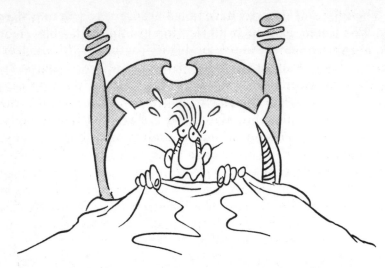

Stress affects us 24 hours a day—even when asleep

Tension headaches

A common presentation of stress which most of us experience from time to time is that of tension headaches. These are caused by contraction in the muscles of the scalp and vary in intensity from mild to severe. They may be experienced all over the head or just in one place, such as the forehead or back of the head. Bright sunlight or movement can make them worse and sometimes they are associated with nausea and vomiting. Tension headaches tend to occur more often in anxious, tense individuals who have difficulty in relaxing.[3]

Migraine headaches

Those who suffer migraine headaches will agree that attacks can be extremely distressing because of their intensity and unpredictability. They are also disabling because not only does the sufferer often have to retire to bed for the duration of the attack, but there is a feeling of general malaise for several days afterwards.

It is widely recognised that migraine can be precipitated by a variety of factors, especially if there is a family history of the disorder. These factors include such diverse things as glare, hot and humid days and certain foods.

Although some patients have noted headaches occurring after they have eaten particular foods (for example, chocolate) or have drunk red wine, the role of dietary factors is still unclear. There is little doubt that some patients are more 'sensitive' to certain foodstuffs than others. It may also be the case that migraine occurs when the chemicals which act as precipitating agents (for example, amines) exceed a threshold in the body.

Many of the foods you eat may contain amines but not cause your migraine, but for instance, a glass of red wine taken with your meal might raise the level of amines above your critical threshold, and it is at this point that a headache will occur.

Stress can also be a significant contributing factor. It has been stated to be 'the most frequent and most important precipitant for common migraine.'[4]

Low back pain

Chronic low back pain is a common symptom and accounts for a great deal of incapacity and absence from work. It often arises from damage to one or more intervertebral discs. These act as cushions between the bones of the spine and when the space between the bones becomes narrowed because of wear and tear on the discs, nerves become trapped at the point where they emerge from the spinal column. The pain that occurs as the result of this structural damage can be aggravated by tension and stress. Sometimes back pain may be present without there being any obvious problems in the spinal column. In such cases the pain is simply caused by constant spasm in the powerful muscles of the lower back. Whatever the cause, reduction of stress and tension will help to lessen or relieve disabling back pain.

The effects of stress on your involuntary systems

The executive headquarters that governs how your body works is the brain. This extremely complex organ has a myriad of functions to perform. Not only does it control the voluntary systems of the body, but it also controls the organs that lie outside your conscious control—the heart, lungs, bowel, sexual organs, kidneys, skin and endocrine glands. The brain controls these two systems by using two quite separate nervous systems. Thus, if you want to move your leg or lift a book, you do so by bringing into action your central nervous system. On the other hand, you do not have the same control over, say, the heart. Try slowing down your heart rate by thinking about it. I doubt if you will succeed without using a technique such as relaxation.

Organs such as the heart, lungs and bowel are controlled by the involuntary or autonomic nervous system. This complex system maintains a constant control over the organs it supplies, speeding up or slowing down their activity as required. The speeding up mechanism is called the sympathetic nervous system and the braking one the parasympathetic. The optimum functioning of an organ depends upon these two divisions being perfectly balanced.

When you experience stress this delicate balance is upset, activity in a particular organ either speeding up or slowing down. With the organ no longer functioning as it should, you soon become aware of certain symptoms or physical signs developing. This interaction of mind and body is often labelled 'psychosomatic'. It is a term that I dislike because it suggests that *you* are responsible for causing your disease or disorder, and clearly this is not so. Invariably you are unaware that the stress you are feeling is the active ingredient or catalyst for the appearance of your symptoms.

Usually stress will manifest its effects through the autonomic nervous system by 'picking out' one organ above the rest. The reasons for this are not entirely clear. We do recognise, however, that some people seem to have an inherited predisposition or 'weakness' to a particular disorder. If, for example, you have a family history of close relatives having raised blood pressure at a relatively early age, this should warn you that you are liable to develop this condition unless you take adequate precautions, and keep your stress levels to a minimum.

The heart of the matter

Over the years, more attention has been focused on the impact of stress on the heart and blood vessels than on any other bodily system. This is probably due to the incapacitating or fatal consequences that stem from a breakdown of functioning in the circulatory system. The heart is a sophisticated pump, and the blood vessels arising from it convey oxygen and nutrients to all parts of the body.

The most common heart disorder is coronary heart disease, caused by the narrowing or blockage of one or more coronary arteries supplying the heart muscles. These muscles, like all others in the body, need a plentiful supply of oxygen in order to function efficiently. If this oxygen supply is diminished it can produce chest pain (angina). If a coronary artery becomes blocked, then it soon leaves a section of heart muscle without a blood supply and that part of the heart muscle dies. This leads to a heart attack, the severity of which will depend on how much muscle has been knocked out of action.

A number of factors are known to increase the likelihood of developing coronary heart disease. Stress is a major factor, especially if one or more of the other heart attack risk factors are present. These include having raised blood pressure (hypertension), smoking, raised blood fats, (cholesterol and lipids), being overweight, and having a family history of coronary heart disease.

Stress can affect the heart and blood vessels in a number of ways. Not only does it cause an actual narrowing or spasm of the coronary arteries but it can also cause blood pressure to rise. It produces these effects through a complex chemical interaction in the body, the net result being that the heart has to work a great deal harder to pump the blood around the body, particularly to the muscles of the heart. If the narrowing of the coronary blood vessels is severe, the heart may find the task too great and respond by producing pain. The result is angina or a heart attack, depending on the extent of the narrowing.

Because of the unequivocal relationship between stress and coronary heart disease, there is clearly a strong case to be made for the integration of stress-reducing techniques into our everyday lives. In this regard, you will see, in Chapters 5 and 8, how self-hypnosis can be an effective preventative technique.

The effects on other blood vessels

Stress can also affect blood vessels other than the heart. Some people notice that whenever the temperature drops, or when they are emotionally upset, their fingers and toes become pale and numb. This condition, known as Raynaud's phenomenon, is caused by spasm in the very fine arteries (arterioles) in the digits.

A more serious effect of stress is its role in raising blood pressure. Normal blood pressure maintains the flow of blood to the tissues of the body, but if it is raised it causes damage to the walls of arteries.

The reasons for someone becoming hypertensive are extremely complex but irrespective of underlying factors such as having an inherited predisposition to it, stress can be a major contributor to the condition. It acts by stimulating the body to release chemicals called catecholamines. These cause blood vessels to become extremely sensitive to blood pressure changes. Blood vessels to muscles dilate and those to the skin constrict. Consequently, the heart has to pump blood against a greater resistance, and hypertension ensues.

You could liken the effects of blood pressure to partially obstructing the end of a garden hose after fully turning on the tap. If there is a weakness in the hose a leak is likely to ensue, or the pipe will rupture at the junction with the tap. Similarly, prolonged elevation of blood pressure can lead to enlargement of the heart, rupture of blood vessels in the brain (a stroke) or bleeding into the eyes (retinal haemorrhage).

The breath of life

As with all our body's normal functions, most of us tend to take our breathing for granted—that is, until we are suddenly afflicted by something that interferes with this easy, rhythmical process. Probably the most distressing breathing disorder, experienced by both children and adults, is asthma. Its frequency and severity may be such that it requires regular hospital admissions, constant medication and leads to chronic ill health. Even in these days of more enlightened medical research and treatment, asthma still proves to be something of a conundrum.

What causes asthma?

Asthma has been defined as 'a psychophysiological disorder . . . [in which there is] an abnormally increased responsiveness of the airways to various stimuli'.[5] This definition suggests that although it is a physical condition, stress and emotion play a major role in its genesis. But why do some people develop asthma and not others? This is not an easy question to answer. Undoubtedly inheritance plays a part in some cases. As to the rest, we do not yet have a complete picture to account for why some of us are more sensitive than others to allergens (for example, pollens, animal hair, dust mites), irritants and infections.

One thing in clear: whether the underlying increased sensitivity of the air passages to allergens or infection is genetically based or not, stress can certainly exacerbate or even precipitate an asthma attack.

How an attack develops

The main feature of an asthma attack is an intermittent and reversible obstruction of the finer airways in the lung. The primary cause of this is a spasm, or contraction, of the tiny muscles surrounding the air passages. Superimposed on this is an inflammation and swelling of the tissues, and the production of excessive mucus. The combined effect of these is to narrow the bronchial passages and make breathing, especially exhalation, extremely laboured and slow. The wheezing, which is a feature of asthma, is caused by air being forced through a spasmed region of the larger airways.

Even though emotional stress has been shown to be a significant factor in either triggering or intensifying an asthmatic attack,[6] not all asthma sufferers are able to associate the two. This is unsurprising for it is often hard to separate cause from effect. Does the emotion cause the attack or is the emotion the result of the episode? It is probably true to say that both views are correct, for as all asthma sufferers will testify, it is an extremely distressing condition. Nevertheless, whichever view one takes, emotional stress *does* lead to a spasm of the bronchial muscles and an increased production of mucus.

Ways of coping with asthma, incorporating self-hypnosis, are outlined in Chapter 8.

Stress and your peptic ulcer

Most of us can recall instances when, faced by some potentially stressful event such as an examination or a job interview, we have felt sick or experienced diarrhoea. In these everyday situations, once the worrying event has passed, the symptoms tend to settle down. The fact that they occur at all indicates how sensitive our abdominal organs are to stress.

A disorder which is often related to stress is peptic ulceration. The ulcers may occur either in the stomach (gastric ulcers), or in the part of the bowel issuing from the stomach (duodenal ulcers). Those with a stress-prone personality are much more likely to develop ulcers, as are those who have a family history of this condition.

The management of peptic ulcers, whether duodenal or gastric, involves taking medication which helps to heal the inflammation, but the stress factor also needs to be dealt with if you are going to encourage their healing. Stress exerts its effect through the autonomic nervous system by causing the stomach and bowel muscles to contract too vigorously. It also creates an inflammation of the lining membrane of these organs so that excessive amounts of digestive juices are produced. Both of these have the effect of irritating the ulcer and can interfere greatly with healing.

The Irritable Bowel Syndrome (IBS)

This distressing bowel condition is far more common than is generally realised, between 50 and 70 per cent of patients with bowel symptoms being said to suffer from it.[7] The symptoms that characterise IBS are abdominal pain, diarrhoea, constipation, rumbling and gurgling of the bowel, rectal bleeding and mucus in the motions. In many people, psychological stress is a significant contributor to the development of IBS.

How stress affects your skin

The skin is by far the largest of the body's organs, and is

obviously the most visible. The skin is greatly influenced by emotional stress and we are all aware of examples of this in everyday life. Some of us, when embarrassed, have a tendency to blush. We have all had frightening experiences that have caused our hair to 'stand on end' and have developed 'goose pimples' when listening to stirring music. Events such as these are transitory in nature and once the stimulus that causes them has passed the skin and its appendages (the hair) return to normal.

But what of the more pathological or abnormal conditions of the skin? A wealth of clinical evidence shows that some skin conditions are caused by emotional stress and, once established, tend to be further intensified by the stress factor.

The skin and the mind: twins

The relationship between the skin and the mind is extremely close, stemming from the earliest days of life, long before the baby is born. Within a week or two of fertilisation taking place, the cell starts to divide into different layers of cells. One of these is called the ectoderm, which simply means the outer layer. Subsequently this layer of cells divides once more. Part remains on the outside of the developing foetus and will form the skin. The other cells migrate inwards and develop into the brain and nervous systems. Thus, although the skin and the brain look nothing alike, they could be considered twins.

It is not surprising therefore, that anything that upsets or stresses the mind is often manifested in the form of a skin lesion. This is why the skin is sometimes labelled 'the mirror of the mind'. In Chapter 8 the treatment of skin disorders through the use of self-hypnosis is outlined.

You and your immune system

One of the most exciting and rewarding areas of study in recent years concerning the mind-body relationship has been in assessing the effects of stress on the body's immunity or defence mechanisms. Arising out of these studies are a number of important findings, the principal one being that stress can have a major suppressant effect on your body's defences.[8] This will result in your being much more susceptible to infections, allergies and even to developing cancer.

The body's defences

Your immune system is a complex surveillance mechanism, the principal function of which is to protect you against invasive or foreign organisms. How well your immune system carries out this function is influenced by two major factors: the level of endocrine substances called corticosteroids in the body, and the number of white cells or lymphocytes in the blood.

Corticosteroids are released by the adrenal glands in the abdomen. These endocrines are essential for the normal functioning of the body, and the pituitary gland in the brain is responsible for delicately controlling levels so that they are neither excessive nor too low. Increased production of corticosteroids has been demonstrated to occur within hours of being exposed to a stressful event. The most important effect of this is to suppress the activity of the body's defence cells, called lymphocytes.[8]

There are two types of defence cells: the B and T lymphocytes. The B cells are produced by the bone marrow and release antibodies which protect your body against bacteria and viruses. T lymphocytes arise from the thymus gland in the neck and have the role of killing cancer cells and certain bacteria and viruses.

Some of the T cells become highly specialised and are called natural killer cells. Their job is to seek out and destroy cancer cells for 'when cancer cells first enter the bloodstream . . .they are highly vulnerable to detection by the immune system'.[5] Since stress serves to suppress the production of these defence cells, it clearly makes you much more vulnerable to infections, allergies and cancer. (In Chapter 8 I deal with the strengthening of the immune system through the use of self-hypnosis.)

STRESS AND YOUR MIND

From the earliest years of our life we are confronted by a whole variety of situations that are potential stressors. The stability of our family life, the need to do well at school and concerns about our work are but a few of the many issues that can gradually create a sense of stress within us. Generally we cope satisfactorily, but even in the strongest of us there may come a time when the sheer amount of this mental strain starts to disturb the way we think and behave.

Perhaps the most surprising thing is not that we do eventually succumb to life's pressures, but rather that we manage to cope with them for as long as we do. In a sense, this happens because our mind becomes progressively desensitised to stress, thereby learning to deal with increasing loads. You could compare this process to one that may confront you when you want to get physically fit. At first, you find that jogging a couple of hundred metres is excessively taxing. With repetition you are able to increase your endurance until finally you are able to cope quite easily with distances which previously would have defeated you.

The breakdown in our mind's coping mechanism can usually be traced to either constant, inescapable stress, or the occurrence of a major traumatic event (known as a superstressor), such as the death of a loved one, loss of a job or severe financial difficulties.

The importance of self-esteem

What happens when your mind becomes overstressed? One of the most significant effects is on your self-esteem. This term is one with which we are all familiar, but ask a cross-section of the public what it means and you are likely to get a wide range of answers.

Some people like to use the term interchangeably with self-confidence, but to do so is not strictly accurate. When we describe someone as having good self-esteem we are recognising that they appreciate their own self-worth and feel accepted by and at ease with others. They cope well with social situations and are comfortable in expressing their own opinions even though their views may be at variance with those of other people.

A person with low self-esteem on the other hand, experiences feelings of worthlessness and all manner of doubts creep into his or her mind—even doubts about being able to perform simple, everyday things satisfactorily. In social situations, such people may feel as though they are 'not good enough' and may wonder why anyone would want to befriend them. Such feelings can carry over into sport and leisure pastimes, serving to further undermine self-belief. If this process goes unchecked, self-esteem continues to plummet: the person becomes more and more isolated from things and people and, inevitably, increasingly stressed.

Undoubtedly some individuals do have better self-esteem than others, for a variety of reasons unassociated with stress. You are born with particular personality traits which can either lead to you being gregarious and outgoing, or shy and introverted. The environment in which you were raised as a child is also likely to influence your subsequent patterns of behaviour. If, for example, you are repeatedly told as a child that 'you are hopeless' at something, you are likely to grow up believing you really *are* hopeless at that thing.

Most of us lead fairly routine lives, restricted by the ever-present demands of daily existence, and rarely exploit our full potential. Nevertheless, we are generally happy and well-adjusted. Once stress intervenes, however, it disturbs the whole balance of life, especially when it undermines self-esteem.

The building of self-esteem through the use of self-hypnosis is covered in some detail in Chapter 5 and, in relation to sport, in Chapter 6.

Impairment of concentration

Difficulty in concentrating is a problem experienced by many and can be a major source of concern, particularly for those who are studying for examinations. But it may also prove to be a hindrance in work situations and other life events.

You may become aware of its presence through having difficulty in remembering things, especially happenings in the recent past. Many attribute this loss of short-term memory to 'getting older' but there is little evidence to support the notion that ageing has a significant effect on memory processes. The most common reason for this apparent loss of recall is that, as we get older, we tend to become selectively disinterested in certain events around us. In other words, we learn to 'switch off' from things which are of no immediate importance.

A more important cause of poor memory is loss of concentration due to stress. In the stressed state the mind becomes overloaded with a variety of intrusive concerns which act to break-up the normal channelling of concentration. The result is a loss of attentional focusing due to our thoughts constantly becoming diverted into areas unconnected with the task in hand.

Sleep problems

Each of us has an innate biological rhythm and sleep is an essential part of our twenty-four hour cycle. If sleep becomes chronically impaired, we feel fatigued and function less effectively in life.

Insomnia can affect people in four ways: there are those who have difficulty falling asleep but subsequently sleep well, those who have no problem getting to sleep but have trouble staying asleep, and those who have both problems. The fourth group wakes an hour or more earlier than usual.

Many things can interfere with one's normal sleep pattern. These include being woken by crying children, loud noise such as traffic, a snoring partner in bed, or having to attend to a family member who is ill. Usually, these disturbances are short term, or one becomes conditioned to them so that they no longer intrude.

More serious causes of insomnia, and ones that persist unless active steps are taken to correct them, are stress and depression. The latter condition will require the help of your physician and no more need be said about it here. Stress, on the other hand, can be a potent cause of sleep disruption and *is* correctable.

It is not difficult to recognise the effects of stress on your sleep pattern. You may feel drowsy and tired on retiring to bed but suddenly your mind is full of unbidden thoughts and worries, ruminating on concerns of the day or forthcoming events. The same pattern can also occur when you awaken at night. This often results in your developing a fear of *not* sleeping and the following chain of events is soon established:

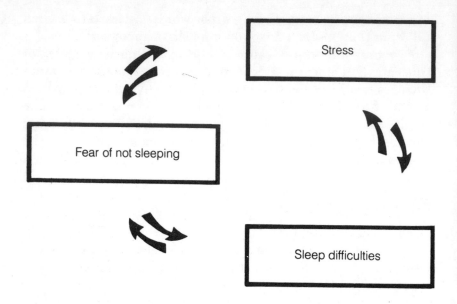

Concern about the need for sleep can become so intense that some resort to taking hypnotic (sleep producing) medication. While useful for the short-term treatment of insomnia, it does have drawbacks. The principal one is that, if taken for a long period of time, there is a distinct possibility of developing a dependency on the drug. Stopping the drug frequently leads to the recurrence of sleep difficulties and, consequently, the person resorts to further medication in order to solve the problem.

Another disturbing aspect of stopping hypnotic medication is excessive dreaming, and this may give you the feeling that you have not slept soundly. Understanding the reason for this more intense dream pattern may allay your concerns. Normal sleep is composed of two distinct phases: dream or rapid eye movement (REM) sleep and non-dream or non-rapid eye movement (NREM) sleep. These processes alternate throughout the night and you can best view dream sleep as the mind's way of releasing the tensions of the day. One effect of hypnotic medication is to partially suppress this phase and thus the mind builds up a deficit of dream sleep. When medication is stopped, the mind attempts to correct the situation by producing excessive amounts of dreams. Be reassured, however, that this is a temporary phenomenon and normal sleep rhythm will soon become reestablished.

The correction of a sleep problem lies in eliminating the stress which is causing it. Not to take steps to deal with the cause would be akin to trying to get rid of smoke without first extinguishing the fire.

Other features of stress

There are other signs, perhaps less obvious, that indicate the presence of stress. On occasions, it can present as feelings of irritability at home, work or in situations such as driving your car. Another common presentation is constant fatigue, often labelled as the 'tired-all-the-time' syndrome. Sometimes there may be a general loss of interest in life events—home, leisure and social activities, and even one's own children. Finally, the stressed person may demonstrate a greater tendency to worry, even relatively insignificant events becoming magnified out of all proportion to their seriousness.

The need to cope

Irrespective of who we are or what we do, we are all going to be faced from time to time with situations that stress us. Many of these events are not necessarily of our making, but whatever their cause, the most important thing from a health point of view is to learn to cope with them.

Our bodies have built-in mechanisms which enable us to cope with short-term stress. The problems start for most people when stress is unremitting. It can then produce some very unpleasant effects on the health of both the body and the mind.

Self-hypnosis enables you to reduce this stress and, more importantly, ensure that it does not recur. But to achieve that sort of control you need to become a devotee to its use. The aim of this book is to show you how to use and enjoy self-hypnosis. You will find in time that it becomes something you look forward to—a pleasant, peaceful interlude in your day.

CHAPTER TWO

HYPNOSIS: THE TRUE PICTURE

You may be wondering why, in this book, we should even consider hypnosis. After all, are we not looking at self-hypnosis and its role in treating stress? The answer is simply that, in order for you to achieve the best results from this therapy, you must, first, be able to understand what happens in the hypnotic state—whether it is induced by someone else (hetero-hypnosis) or by yourself (self-hypnosis). Heterohypnosis is by convention known as hypnosis.

More is known of hypnosis than self-hypnosis. This may be due to the fact that since its early days it has excited more interest, both from researchers and clinicians. Self-hypnosis does not easily lend itself to research study: of 1200 articles on hypnosis published in major journals between 1958 and 1973, only twenty-four dealt with self-hypnosis.[9] This is not to say that self-hypnosis is of lesser importance, however, for clearly this is not the case. The use of self-hypnosis allows *you* to take charge of your own destiny, in effect to become your own therapist.

One of the major bones of contention amongst clinicians and researchers is whether you need to first experience hypnosis before learning the art of self-hypnosis. Some claim it is desirable[10] whilst others maintain that you can learn self-hypnosis once you know what procedures to use and how best to apply them. This is the view that I favour, but for you to be able to hypnotise yourself effectively, it is extremely important that, first, you should have an understanding of what happens in the hypnotic state.

Mesmerism

Although there is evidence that trance states were used in healing as far back as Babylonian days, the real history of hypnosis starts in the mid-eighteenth century with a flamboyant Paris physician, Dr. Franz Mesmer. He discovered that he could induce a trance state, labelled by him as mesmerism or animal magnetism, by having his patients stand around a wooden tub called a baquet, which was filled with iron filings and water. Each patient grasped a metal rod protruding from the tub and, in response to suggestions from Mesmer, they experienced 'crises'. When they came out of these crises, it is reported that they were cured of their various ailments. The whole procedure was carried out in a darkened room, Mesmer adding to the air of mystique by appearing in a purple cloak, sometimes quietly playing the piano whilst his patients were undergoing treatment. Mesmer firmly believed that it was his presence that was a major ingredient in creating the trance state in his patients.

The work of Mesmer aroused a great deal of controversy in the medical circles of his day and this led to his being investigated by two Commissions of Enquiry set up by Louis XVI, equivalent to our present-day Royal Commissions. One of the commissions included such notables as Bailly the astronomer, Lavoisier the chemist, Dr Guillotin (who achieved notoriety for something far removed from healing), and the American Ambassador, Benjamin Franklin. After much deliberation, they decided that there was little substance to Mesmer's work and ascribed its curative effects to imagination and suggestion. This was intended to dismiss its value as a therapy, but now, two hundred years later, we realise these two processes form an essential part of all hypnotic and self-hypnotic treatment.

The start of the hypnotic era

The next major step occurred in the 1840s, centred on a

Manchester surgeon, Dr James Braid. Initially Braid viewed Mesmer's therapy with scepticism, but when he put the treatment to the test he was impressed by the beneficial effects it had on some of his patients. Unlike Mesmer, however, Braid determined that the changes brought about in his patients were not due to the skills of the operator but, rather, to those of the subject. Here you can see the beginnings of self-hypnosis as a therapy.

Braid was astute enough to observe the importance of getting his patients to focus on one idea at a time. This focusing of attention is still recognised as being one of the prime requirements for achieving a disengaged state of mind. The term 'disengaged' simply refers to the mind becoming still and quiet—a state in which it is free of thoughts and intrusions.

However, Braid made the mistake of labelling this state 'hypnosis', derived from the Greek word 'hypnos', meaning sleep. He did so because he believed that patients experienced sleep, which we now know to be entirely false. To be fair to Braid, he later realised his mistake and attempted to re-label it 'monoideism' (one single thought). Unfortunately, the term hypnosis was too firmly entrenched, and over a century later we are still struggling with this controversial connotation.

Since Braid's seminal studies, interest in hypnosis by the medical and psychological world has waxed and waned. Interest has been maintained by the enthusiasm of a large number of notable workers, its acceptance by modern-day medicine being assured when, in the 1950s, the British Medical Association and the American Medical Association issued statements supporting its usefulness as a form of therapy. When we consider the number of doctors, dentists and psychologists throughout the world who use hypnosis in their practice, it is easy to see that it has come of age.

What is hypnosis?

Misconceptions about hypnosis abound. Many of these fallacies can be traced back to the unfortunate use of hypnosis as a form of entertainment on stage and television. Literary works such as George Du Maurier's *Trilby* have served to fuel these faulty impressions.

The best way to view hypnosis is as a state of intense relaxation and concentration, in which the mind becomes disengaged or detached from everyday cares and concerns. In this relaxed state the mind is best able to respond to suggestions and imagery (mental pictures). It can, as it were, focus on the things you want to change and on the ways you can best go about changing them, free from anxious thoughts. It is almost as though that state of inner mental peace allows you the opportunity to fit back into place those pieces of the mind's jigsaw puzzle which have been disrupted by stress or anxiety.

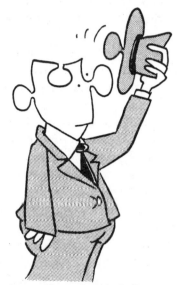

A relaxed state allows the mind's jigsaw puzzle to fit
neatly together

Some people like to think of hypnosis as a state of altered consciousness. In that you feel more relaxed and peaceful, can experience pleasant feelings of heaviness, floating or a sense of detachment from things around you, consciousness is certainly altered. I do, however, get a little concerned by the term for it may signify to some that they are going to experience sensations and responses over which they have little or no control. This is entirely incorrect, and I prefer to think of hypnosis (and self-hypnosis) as an *alternative* state of consciousness. It is a creative experience because it provides

25

you with the opportunity to use imagery and suggestion, in a state free from anxiety, so that you can gradually modify your behaviour problems.

Let us now look at the most common misconceptions that people tend to have about hypnosis.

The sleep notion

So entrenched are the theatrical connotations of the term 'hypnosis' that the mention of it immediately engenders, in the minds of many, an image of a man with a fixed, penetrating gaze swinging a pocket-watch and murmuring such phrases as 'You are now going deeply asleep'. To anyone unfamiliar with hypnosis, it certainly does seem that the hypnotised subject is in a state of sleep. They imagine that if they should be hypnotised they will be unable to hear anything and be unaware of their surroundings.

Hypnosis, in fact, is as distinct from sleep as day is from night. Far from being a state of unconsciousness, it is one of intense relaxation in which you are encouraged to concentrate on one thought or idea at a time. Imagine you are asleep. Obviously, in this state there would be little point in making any suggestions to you. You would simply not respond to them. Compare this with hypnosis and self-hypnosis, where the mind is extremely responsive to suggestion. For those with a more scientific turn of mind, the technique of electroencephalography (EEG), which measures tracings of the brain's activity, has unequivocally demonstrated a clear difference between sleep and hypnosis.

Will I lose control?

When you view someone being hypnotised and 'performing' on stage, you get the impression that the subject is very much under the control of the hypnotist. The hypnotist may suggest to subjects that they will cluck like chickens, for example, whenever he clicks his fingers. When they do respond to the signal this gives casual observers the idea that, even if they wished to, they are unable to resist. Fortunately, this is not the case.

If you were to be hypnotised, you *could* resist if you so desired. The reasons for your compliance would have a lot to do with the expectations you have when you go up on stage. You would expect to be asked to perform. You may also believe that you will be unable to resist, but if you were told to do something embarrassing or morally unacceptable, you would have no qualms about refusing. In fact, you would probably come out of hypnosis spontaneously. In other words, you would only comply because you felt comfortable in doing so, not because the hypnotist had control over your mind.

The hypnotist acts purely as a guide or leader. The hypnotic relationship is best understood as a cooperative exercise[11] in which the therapist acts as the coach. As in any team situation, the coach can suggest things to you, but you do not necessarily have to comply. If you have a strong belief in your mentor, however, you are much more likely to respond to suggestions given to you. This is the essence of the therapist-patient relationship.

Hand-in-hand with the faulty belief that you have no control over what you do goes the fear that you will disclose things you have no wish to reveal. An aspect of this fear is the expectation that hypnosis (and self-hypnosis) will cause you to spontaneously uncover past traumatic events—ones that you have no desire to recall because of their unpleasantness. Although hypnosis can be used therapeutically to 'free up' past memories that may be acting as a source of many of your anxieties, this can only take place if you are agreeable. In a treatment situation, a therapist usually seeks the patient's acquiescence before embarking on this procedure. If you are unwilling to engage in such an exercise the same mental blocking processes will operate in hypnosis as do in your everyday life.

But I can remember all you said

This is what people commonly say, in some surprise, when they discuss their experiences after their first session of hypnosis. The misconception that you will remember nothing of what has happened also has its roots in mesmerism. Some early workers noticed that subjects, like sleepwalkers, had no recollection of anything they had said or done when they came out of trance. Because of this, they assumed that amnesia was one of the hall-marks of mesmerism.

It is faintly possible that a small minority of hypnotic subjects *can* spontaneously experience the phenomenon of loss of memory for events in hypnosis—labelled as posthypnotic amnesia. A considerable amount of research has been directed towards the issue of posthypnotic amnesia, however, and has shown that, in the majority of people, amnesia will only occur if appropriate suggestions are made to the hypnotised subject. For all intents and purposes, you can assume that after hypnosis, or self-hypnosis, you will be able to remember everything that has been said or that you experienced, making allowance for the normal process of forgetting, which can affect us all.

I felt I wanted to move

Many people believe that they have to remain absolutely still in hypnosis or self-hypnosis for fear of 'breaking the spell'. You may have an itch on the end of your nose and desperately want to scratch it, or you might feel uncomfortable in a certain position, but rather than take appropriate steps to correct the situation, you exert as much will-power as possible to keep the urge in check.

However, changing position or scratching your nose is less likely to interfere with your hypnotic or self-hypnotic state than if you try to resist such urges. Concern about not doing these things will prove far more intrusive to your relaxation and mental disengagement than actually doing them. So the maxim is, if you have an itch, scratch it.

Perhaps I should try harder

From earliest childhood we are invoked to try hard in everything we do, the idea being that the harder we try, the better we will become. Generally, we cannot argue with this thesis: if we study hard for examinations, work hard in our job or practice our sport, then it follows that we can expect to achieve greater success. But if you approach hypnosis or self-hypnosis with the belief that you should *try* to relax, you will probably be disappointed with your results. This is because hypnosis involves *letting things happen* rather than trying to make them happen.

When your therapist takes you through the induction or disengagement procedures of hypnosis, or, in the case of self-hypnosis, you take yourself through these procedures, the aim is to gradually quieten your conscious mind—to help it become less involved. But if you *try* to achieve these things, you will be bringing your conscious mind back into operation. The answer lies in approaching hypnosis and self-hypnosis with the attitude that you are just going to let whatever happens happen. Only in this way will you experience the sense of complete quietness of mind that characterises these techniques.

Will the good effects last?

One of the earlier charges laid at the door of hypnosis was that its effects were temporary. The doctors who held this view were those who were schooled in the therapeutic approach of psychoanalysis. They believed that it was far too rapid in producing its beneficial effects and did not help a patient get to the core of the problem, something that they felt was necessary if treatment was to be effective.

Over the years, a gradual transition has taken place with regard to the processes that are used in helping a person learn to manage problems such as stress. Instead of trying to identify events in the dim and distant past which might have had some bearing on present problems, there has developed another approach—that of behaviour therapy.

This therapy is designed to help you cope more satisfactorily with here-and-now things in your life. If, for example, you have a phobia of spiders, you are taught to cope with this by being gradually introduced to the feared object until you are able to tolerate it with ease. This process, known as desensitisation, can be employed effectively in hypnosis and self-hypnosis using mental imagery.

Behaviour therapy can help you, too, to restructure your 'wrong' thinking. Negative thinking can cause you to become anxious and stressed and will serve to undermine your self-esteem. In other words, think bad, feel bad. The aim of therapy, especially when it is incorporated into hypnosis or self-hypnosis, is to help you change the way you think so that you think good, feel good.

With the wider acceptance of behaviour therapy, and the realisation that hypnosis is a valuable arena in which to integrate this approach, has come an acknowledgement that the therapeutic effects of hypnosis and self-hypnosis are anything but temporary in nature.

There are occasions in our lives when stress can become so great that we fear that we will be unable to cope, either at home or at work. Hypnosis and self-hypnosis can change all this. Their effects are strangely paradoxical. While many of the benefits seem to happen unconsciously, the changes that do occur can be quite dramatic in their speed and intensity.

There is little doubt that the daily use of self-hypnosis will ensure that new patterns of relaxed behaviour become integrated into your life. It will provide you with all the skills necessary to change the things you want to change—your thinking, the manner in which you react to people and situations, and the way you feel about yourself.

Once these changes start to occur, they will become self-perpetuating. You will realise you can cope with what once seemed formidable problems, and so you will approach other situations with far greater expectations of success. The therapeutic effects of hypnosis and self-hypnosis are undoubtedly ongoing and permanent.

Your motivation for change

The two main factors that will determine how effective hypnosis (and also self-hypnosis) will be for you are, first, how much you *really* want to change your behaviour and attitudes and, second, how involved you become in your treatment. What we are touching on here is your motivation—to be more precise, your unconscious motivation—to get better. In other words, *you* are the essential catalyst in therapy. For although you may feel that you are weary of having to constantly face up to your stress-related problems and consequently want to unburden yourself of them, your unconscious mind can sometimes prove to be devious and unhelpful. It is almost as though it prefers to cling on to known behaviours, even if they interfere with peace of mind and quality of life.

Your decision to beat your stress problems must take into account the fact that, although hypnotic and self-hypnotic treatment is relatively rapid in action, it will still need your constant involvement. Unless you are prepared to commit yourself to using self-hypnosis on a day-to-day basis, you are unlikely to achieve all the benefits you should.

Most endeavours if life require effort of some sort if you wish to get the most out of them. If your goal is getting physically fit, for example, this will entail your exercising on a daily basis. Similarly, mental fitness calls for the same dedication. Before you embark on this path to attaining inner mental peace and a stress-free existence, first ask yourself if you are prepared to devote the time and effort necessary for doing the relaxation exercises.

Many start off using hypnosis and self-hypnosis with a great flurry of enthusiasm, only to soon lose momentum. They end up feeling disappointed with themselves and the therapy because it has failed to live up to their expectations. For this reason, perhaps the first thing you should do is to sit down and ponder on the problems you have. Think about how much they are interfering with your quality of life and how much better you would feel if they were replaced by more relaxed attitudes and behaviours. Doing this will help provide you with the impetus you need, not only to get started but also to build these relaxation exercises into your lifestyle.

I'm too strong-willed

All of us like to think of ourselves as strong-willed individuals who are not easily induced to do things which are in any way contrary to our own wishes. Not surprisingly, anything that is perceived as lessening our sense of control is viewed with caution and, at times, frank suspicion.

It has been my experience that some people have considerable difficulty going into hypnosis because of the fear that they will lose control. As has already been stated, there is no loss of control. You are *always* in charge and you can come out of hypnosis if ever you feel the need to do so.

Another, related, misconception is that only weak-minded,

gullible people can be hypnotised. People with such a view erect a variety of unconscious barriers which effectively prevent them from going into the hypnotic state, but there is certainly no justification for this notion.

People do, however, have varying degrees of hypnotic potential—a factor called hypnotisability. A small percentage of the population can experience deep hypnosis: more will be said about this special group a little later. A much larger group are moderately hypnotisable and another small group can only achieve a light plane of hypnosis. Unfortunately, there is a fourth group who have little or no hypnotic ability at all. As we will see, this is not because they are actively resisting or being uncooperative, but results from factors entirely outside their control.

What makes a good hypnotic subject?

Your ability to achieve hypnosis, and therefore self-hypnosis, depends upon a mixture of characteristics, some of which are inborn. The most obvious one is that you must be willing to experience this relaxed state of mind. Even those who have good hypnotic potential can resist if they have the mind to do so. This most commonly occurs because of a fear, born of ignorance, of what is likely to happen to them when hypnosis is induced. In order to circumvent these fears, a therapist will invariably go to great lengths to allay a person's concerns about hypnosis before embarking on treatment. This is a very necessary procedure, for without it the subject may find it extremely hard to 'let go' of tensions, concerns and apprehension.

Good concentration

Another feature of good hypnotic subjects is that they are invariably intelligent and have excellent powers of concentration. It would seem that people who have gone through some form of disciplined training and regimentation in their life, especially with their studies, are more susceptible to hypnosis. All of this is contrary to popular belief that weak-minded and gullible people are more easily hypnotised. In fact, they tend to make rather poor hypnotic subjects owing to their inability to concentrate for any length of time on what is being asked of them.

The importance of imagination

You constantly tap into your imaginative ability, sometimes without even being aware of it. A good example of this is when a friend has told you about a holiday, describing a beach, country scene or old mansion they visited, and you visualised it, even without having been there. When you do this, you use your imaginative powers to convert a word scene into a visual picture.

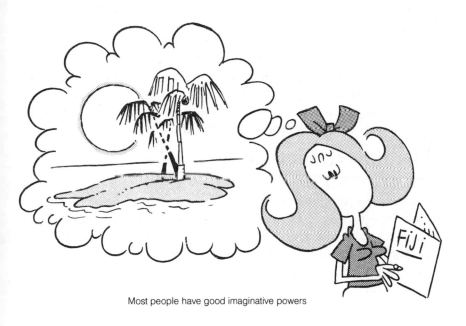

Most people have good imaginative powers

We use these powers in other ways too. Fantasy and daydreaming can be important in our lives by allowing us to temporarily escape from reality into imagined situations and events which are not necessarily achievable in real life. The imagery associated with fantasy and daydreaming is not unlike that experienced in hypnosis and self-hypnosis, except that in these states it is deliberately induced by the therapist or yourself. Occasionally it can occur quite spontaneously and when it does you will find it enriching and therapeutically beneficial.

The power of imagery varies from individual to individual. Some people seem to have an enormous capacity for imaginative involvement [12] and this ability is often closely related to a person's artistic nature. Singers, musicians, painters and writers tend to have rich imaginations. Elite sportspeople too, invariably possess the ability to summon up strong images.

It is not just coincidence that such people have a great capacity for imaginative involvement. They all have one feature in common—the ability to 'lose themselves' in their art or sport. Because of this, they can become so absorbed in what they are doing that they lose all track of things around them. This intensity of involvement may be the prime reason for their success.

Subjects with this great capacity for imaginative involvement are invariably excellent hypnotic subjects because of their natural predisposition to become totally absorbed in whatever they do. Disengaging from intrusive thoughts and happenings around them (one of the prerequisites for achieving hypnosis) is a normal, everyday experience for them.

The inheritance factor

A final factor which may decide how deeply you can go into hypnosis is one that you inherit, especially from your mother's side of the family.[13] However, the non-hypnotisable subject is relatively rare and most of us *are* hypnotisable to some degree or other. In the long term what matters most is not so much your degree of hypnotisability but rather, how you use the talents you do possess.

SELF-HYPNOSIS, AND HOW TO INDUCE IT

Throughout the history of hypnosis, most of the research and clinical interest has centred around the interaction between the person being hypnotised (the subject) and the person doing the hypnotising (the hypnotiser). When you are treated in hypnosis, the therapist's role is to help you experience the hypnotic state and, whilst in that state, to treat your problems in the manner best suited to you. Unquestionably, this treatment can be most valuable for you, but there is also a need for you to learn certain techniques of your own, which I like to call skills. Most doctors and therapists emphasise to their patients the importance of learning to use these procedures. In other words, they stress the importance of you becoming your own therapist. When you induce hypnosis on your own, without the involvement of anyone else, you are using self-hypnosis.

How does self-hypnosis differ from hypnosis?

How, then, does heterohypnosis differ from self-hypnosis? Essentially, they are much the same state. They employ similar techniques, their therapeutic uses are similar and the way you bring yourself out of both states is much the same. The main difference experienced by those who have experienced both hypnosis and self-hypnosis concerns the depth of relaxation. People frequently comment on the fact that their feeling of relaxation appears to be less deep during self-hypnosis. This often concerns them, since they believe that either they are not doing it properly or that the benefits are not going to be as great because of this apparent lack of depth.

Indeed it *is* true that the depth of hypnosis you experience when you induce it in yourself is not as great as when someone else does it for you. The most likely reason for this is that your conscious mind has to take over as therapist and guide in self-hypnosis. It has to play an active role throughout. Contrast this with hypnosis where the therapist acts as the guide and where the conscious mind is encouraged to play as little a part as possible.

The problem of thought focusing

Another factor that may account for the lesser depth that appears to occur in self-hypnosis is the difficulty that most people experience, especially in the early stages, in keeping their mind concentrated on the procedures themselves. Even in our everyday life, most of us find difficulty in focusing our mind on one thing for any length of time without some distracting thought creeping in. But it is essential to empty the mind of competing thoughts if you are to achieve any significant depth of disengagement. In hypnosis, even though you have the voice of the hypnotist to concentrate upon, it can be exceedingly difficult for you to keep your mind on what is being said or on the sensations you are experiencing. The mind is prone to becoming caught up in mundane thoughts, say work matters or what you are going to cook for dinner.

Given that this happens easily enough when you have the words of the therapist to focus upon, it is not difficult to understand why you should find it hard to disengage mentally when *you* are the guide. And the more tense and anxious you are, the harder this focusing process tends to become. As one of my patients so graphically put it 'Whenever I settle down to use my self-hypnosis, I seem to have the mind of an agitated monkey!' I will describe a little later the ways in which you can learn to bring your wayward mind under control.

Your mental hammer

Do not be concerned if at first you find it hard to achieve a deep sense of relaxation and disengagement using self-hypnosis. You will still find that the benefits you experience are considerable. Depth of relaxation is not all-important. When you visit your doctor for hypnotherapy, it is as though he is able to hit your problems very hard using a large mental hammer. On your own, the mental hammer you use is a little smaller but, to offset this, you can hit the target problems more frequently and so achieve the same end result.

Another reason why you should not be concerned about the issue of depth is that, in self-hypnosis, you will achieve a much greater breadth of experience.[10] One advantage of this is that you will be able to develop your imagery processes to a greater extent than if you were hypnotised by a therapist. It is almost as if nature makes up for the lack of depth by broadening your mental scope.

Myths and misconceptions

Just as hypnosis tends to have its full complement of myths and misconceptions, as discussed in Chapter 2, so too does self-hypnosis. Concerns about the techniques are not often voiced by those who wish to learn them, but if their unspoken questions are left unanswered, they can serve as unconscious 'blocks.' A person may be unable to 'let go', for fear of some devilish unsought thing occurring when he or she is in the self-hypnotic state. Often there are also fears that they may inadvertently explore earlier parts of their life which may have been traumatic. This is a process known as regression. The folklore of hypnosis abounds with stories of people who have been regressed to earlier parts of their life in order to re-experience them.

Can you spontaneously regress?

In hypnosis, where the person is being guided by a therapist, it *is* possible for some people to be regressed, but such a process is always carried out thoughtfully and carefully and under strict control of the therapist. In such instances the hypnotic state is used as an uncovering mechanism so that any memories which are unearthed can be used to help patients deal effectively with the problem that is bothering them. The uncovered material is usually outside conscious awareness and, by having a better understanding or insight into it, the patient is able to cope more effectively with it. Therapists call this process reintegration.

There is no evidence to show that regression occurs spontaneously in self-hypnosis. For one thing, true regression (or revivication) only occurs in those who are capable of entering very deep hypnosis. These people are the highly hypnotisable group, which only constitutes 5 to 10 per cent of the population, and even for them the depth of trance achieved in self-induction is unlikely to enable them to explore past experiences. In any case, the conscious mind acts very much like a watchdog and is unlikely to allow any process to occur which would be detrimental to health and peace of mind.

Another concern voiced by some is whether they are likely to start revealing their innermost secrets to others whilst in self-hypnosis. This is a complete myth. Self-hypnosis is generally practised alone, but even if you did it in the presence of others, you would not start to reveal your innermost thoughts. Self-hypnosis is not some form of truth serum.

Can I bring myself out of self-hypnosis?

'How do I know that I can come out of the trance when I want to?' ask some of my patients, or 'Is there a possibility that I may be stuck in it?' The answer to both of these questions is that you can bring self-hypnosis to a close whenever you wish. There is nothing to stop you just opening your eyes, but generally you use a counting technique to gradually lighten your trance before opening your eyes. By doing this you avoid the heavy, semi-sleepy stage that results for a short time, if you come out of self-hypnosis too abruptly.

What if I go to sleep?

There is also the question of what happens if you inadvertently fall asleep. This can happen easily because of the feelings of complete inner peace you have in self-hypnosis. The main reason for guarding against it is that, once you go to sleep, you are no longer actively involved in your therapy.

If you do go to sleep, however, nothing untoward will happen to you, and you will awaken spontaneously after a short while feeling quite refreshed. In fact, self-hypnosis is sometimes deliberately employed as a peaceful interlude and preparation for sleep by those who suffer from insomnia.

It can be seen then that, as with hypnosis, there is no cause for your having fears or concerns about using self-hypnosis. It is a perfectly safe procedure and one in which *you* remain in control. It is the fear of loss of control that really bothers some people. But would you fear loss of control if you closed your eyes for a while and daydreamed? I doubt it very much. In the same way, you can explore self-hypnosis confident that your mind is under control even if you do feel detached or disengaged from things around you and from your cares and concerns.

Why should I use self-hypnosis?

To provide an answer to this question is to provide the linchpin for the whole book.

In Chapter 1 I talked of stress and anxiety being major problems in today's world. Each of us experiences stress to some degree every day. While sometimes the things that are stressful act as a stimulus to us (eustress), generally they interfere with our health, peace of mind, efficiency and enjoyment of the world around us. Some of these stress-inducing factors, or stressors as they are called, are associated directly with us; others lie outside our control. Reaction to stressors varies enormously from individual to individual, and what may prove highly stressful to one person may act as a stimulus and challenge to another.

I am often asked 'Why should I be stressed? After all, I have a happy home life, my job is secure and I have a good income.' In view of all these features, it may indeed be difficult, at first, to understand why such a person is stressed. The answer lies in two major factors: inherited makeup and environment. Just as we inherit certain characteristics from our parents or forebears, such as eye colour and physical build, so too do we inherit predispositions to certain physical and mental disorders. Stress is one of these.

Coupled with these inherited tendencies are environmental factors. From birth we are influenced constantly by things that are happening around us—by our home environment, school, work and personal life situations. Without necessarily being aware of it, we respond strongly to these environmental factors, especially when young. A great deal of our present behaviour was shaped by the reactions of those around us. Significant people in our lives act as models and we tend to shape ourselves and our behaviours on what we observe and hear. Most of this goes on outside conscious awareness—it is involuntary. If we are surrounded constantly by an anxious and tense environment, this will frequently lead to our becoming tense and stressed.

The importance of mental ease

It is interesting to see how 'stress' and 'anxiety' have become common parlance and are frequently used interchangeably. As I discussed in Chapter 1, both can be viewed as states of mental overload, which often lead to dis-ease (lack of ease) in the body. The aim of treatment, therefore, must be to establish a state of mental *ease*.

To establish this state of psychological ease you must not only be able to produce a sense of mental and bodily relaxation (although this is a very necessary prerequisite), but also be able to gradually modify those unacceptable patterns of behaviour that have occurrred *as the result* of stress and anxiety. I emphasise the word 'gradually' because it is simply not possible to rid yourself of poor behaviours in a short period. It takes time and effort to do so and you should be prepared to use a great deal of repetition of stress-control techniques if you wish to develop sound coping skills. Once these skills are acquired, they will enable you to handle a wide variety of situations in life with ease.

What I am suggesting, in other words, is that to change for the better, the ways you react to particular events or stressors in your life (what psychologists term behaviour modification), is an accumulative process. The more you work on it the better it will become.

How does self-hypnosis help?

I have spent a considerable time discussing the basis of anxiety and stress in órder to provide you with a rationale for applying self-hypnosis. I do not see this technique as some form of magic wand which will miraculously change your whole approach to life so that you become a relaxed, problem-free person. To view self-hypnosis in this way would not only be inappropriate, but also quite unrealistic.

I like to consider self-hypnosis as a means by which you can set aside a small part of each day in order to acquire a relaxed, disengaged state of mind and use that state in a constructive way to re-form the things that bother you. It provides a peaceful environment in which problems of the day can be resolved through the use of coping suggestions and mental imagery. As a patient so delightfully expressed it, 'I can't wait to get home to have an appointment with myself.'

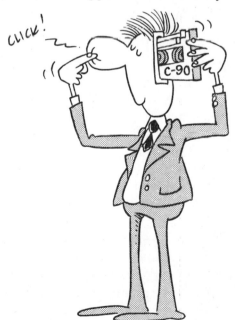

The aim of self-hypnosis is to record a new set of messages on your mental tape

One of the best ways of looking at self-hypnosis is to imagine the mind as a mental cassette recording on which, in the past, a whole series of messages and material have been recorded. Unfortunately, however, not all these recordings have been positive ones, some of them having turned out to be detrimental to your health and well-being. In self-hypnosis you are aiming to re-record a new set of messages on your mental tape. By doing this, you will gradually erase the old, unwanted material. Unlike a normal cassette recorder, the mind does not possess the ability to erase and re-record in one session and can only do it over a period of time. Hence the need for repetition. If you are to succeed you must see self-hypnosis as an ongoing technique.

Self-hypnosis and your body

The human body is a wonderfully sensitive, complicated and powerful creation. It consists of a complex array of organs, systems and endocrines which are controlled through the brain and nervous system. This is why the absence of brain functioning is used routinely as an indicator of the cessation of life. Built into our system is a very important response known as the fight-or-flight mechanism. It is not peculiar to man but forms an integral part of all animal and bird life. In effect, it is a survival mechanism, for it allows us to deal with dangerous or life-threatening adversaries by either adopting a defensive stance or taking flight from the threat.

In conditions of threat, the human body releases large amounts of chemicals called adrenaline, noradrenaline and norepinephrine which stimulate muscles and other bodily organs to greater activity. This allows us to take the appropriate action of standing our ground and fighting, or quickly running away.

As essential and, at times, necessary as this process is, it is intended as a short-term response. What has been demonstrated is that in anxious people the body continues to create increased levels of these chemicals which, in turn, can have a damaging effect on certain organs such as the blood vessels. It can, for instance, lead to an elevation of blood pressure and cause the heart to work excessively hard. It would be similar to you driving your car with the choke constantly pulled out.

You may drive faster for a while but in the long term, you would use up more petrol and cause significant damage to the car's engine. Self-hypnosis can provide you with a means of pushing in the choke and thereby decreasing the blood levels of these potentially damaging chemical substances.

Are your tranquillisers really necessary?

Many people find the many stressors of life intolerable and resort to the use of medication as a means of coping, most frequently taking drugs called benzodiazepines. There is a whole family of these tranquilliser drugs and they can play a valuable short-term role in helping people cope with tension and anxiety.

Unfortunately, however, some people continue to take tranquillisers over a long period, and may become dependent, finding that, unless they have their daily 'fix', they cannot cope even with simple everyday events. Not surprisingly, many are disturbed by being reliant on some form of tablet in order to see the day through. If you are in such a situation, you will find that the daily use of self-hypnosis will provide a valuable alternative to the drugs, enabling you to develop your own inner control over stress. Being free from having to take tranquillisers can be a most fulfilling feeling and will do a great deal to help reinforce your self-esteem and confidence.

One cautionary note: if you are planning to stop taking tranquillisers, it is vital that you do so in a gradual way. It has been shown that the human brain and nervous system is extremely sensitive to even minute doses of these drugs. So be kind to yourself and taper them off over a long period of time. By doing this, you will be less likely to experience any severe withdrawal effects.

Choosing an ideal situation

A belief widely held by many is that self-hypnosis is a meditative state which can *only* be achieved in a peaceful environment. This view, although partially true, has no real basis in fact, for it is possible to use self-hypnosis in a wide variety of situations. If you suffer from a fear of flying, for example, it is perfectly feasible to use it whilst you are sitting in an aeroplane. Nevertheless, in the *initial* stages of learning to use self-hypnosis it is desirable to achieve the most favourable conditions possible. As you become more skilled you will find that you can, in fact, use the technique wherever you wish.

When you first set out to use self-hypnosis, try to find as quiet a place at home as you can—one where there is little likelihood of being interrupted by other members of the household, by family pets, or distracted by outside noises such as traffic. It is helpful to disconnect the telephone for a while, for you may otherwise find that it has the uncanny knack of ringing when you are in the middle of your relaxation session!

Closing out distractions

The major difficulties that everyone encounters when first using self-hypnosis are the focusing of attention and the removal of all sorts of internally-generated thoughts. While this may not seem much of a problem, unfortunately, when you close your eyes and embark on achieving a relaxed, still mind, something devilish seems to happen. Suddenly, a whole host of disconnected thoughts (inner distractions) comes rushing into your mind unbidden, and you are then faced with the uphill task of trying to get rid of them. The presence of *outside* distractions will also add to your burden, which may, in some cases, then prove unmanageable.

The best way to deal with unavoidable outside distractions is to use them to your advantage rather than trying to fight them off. If you adopt the positive approach of saying to yourself 'As I hear the sounds of . . .[for example, children playing in the street], they will take me deeper and deeper into my relaxed state,' your mind will focus much less on them. This approach will cause the sounds to blend into the background.

Do you sit or lie down?

The quietest room for self-hypnosis is quite frequently the bedroom. Although you may think the bed is the most obvious place to relax, do not be tempted to use it. You will have become conditioned to associate bed with sleep, and in a state of extreme relaxation it may prove very difficult to prevent yourself from falling asleep. This, of itself, does no harm, but it does interfere with self-hypnosis.

I would recommend that you use a comfortable lounge chair or lie on a blanket or sponge-rubber yoga mat. If you utilise a chair, make sure that it is high enough in the back to support your head. If you feel more comfortable with your legs elevated, use either a footstool or another chair.

When is the best time?

There can be no hard and fast rules about the most suitable time of the day to use self-hypnosis, for it is generally a matter of when time is available. Many of us have busy work and home schedules. Although it is acceptable to do it at any time, it is preferable not to leave it too late in the day because of the difficulty in concentrating when you are tired. Allow time to complete the session and have a few minutes pause before resuming your activities.

Two other issues are sometimes raised by my patients: should you try to do it at roughly the same time each day, and is it better to avoid using it after a meal? The answer to the first question is that you would probably find it easier to apply self-hypnosis if it is performed each day at approximately the same time. Because your mind can become easily conditioned to a particular pattern of behaviour, if you use your relaxation procedures at a particular time, they tend to become easier and easier to implement.

The second question is not so easy to answer. Many texts on hypnosis and relaxation emphasise that the post-meal phase if to be avoided. I have yet to find any scientific evidence to justify this belief and, for this reason, hold no strong views on it.

THE INDUCTION OF SELF-HYPNOSIS

There are a great many ways of leading yourself into self-hypnosis, just as there are many pathways into hypnosis. Some involve relaxation techniques, others the use of imagery. All, however, aim at the attainment of a quiet, relaxed mind. How you achieve that peaceful mind and body is not important, as long as the procedures suit you.

I like to consider self-hypnosis as being in two parts or phases: the induction phase and the therapeutic phase. The induction phase is necessary in order to prepare the mind—to relax it to the point where it is sensitive or open to suggestions and imagery. Having achieved a relaxed, sensitive mind, you can then apply certain techniques in the therapeutic phase to help you modify those things that you would like to change in yourself. The induction phase could be seen as digging your mind's garden; the therapeutic phase as planting that garden. More will be said of the latter phase in Chapter 4.

Closing your eyes

The purpose of this first step is to enable you to shut out as many distracting stimuli as possible and thereby make it easier to lose yourself into a state of detachment from things around you. Generally it is sufficient to simply close your eyes. Some therapists recommend staring at a small point or target until the eyes become fatigued and close quite naturally. Others suggest an eye roll technique in which the person rolls the eyes upwards and, whilst maintaining the eyes in that position, slowly brings the eyelids down until they are closed.[14]This is a useful procedure since it oftens leads to a slight feeling of detachment. Why this occurs is not entirely clear, but there does seem to be a correlation between a person's ability to roll up the eyes and their hypnotisability. Although it is a useful technique, it is probably better learnt under the guidance of a therapist.

Deepening your relaxation

Once your eyes are closed, you can then call upon a large number of techniques in order to deepen your state of bodily and mental relaxation. You may find, at first, that it is relatively easy to achieve physical relaxation but considerably harder to relax your mind. If this occurs, you should not feel unduly concerned. Your mind is far more open to distraction than you realise and to bring that distractability under control needs considerable practice and patience.

The procedures that I will describe are designed to help you train the mind to relax and focus down on one single thought at a time. It is useful to use a number of procedures so that you can achieve a deep level of mental disengagement. These can be classified under the headings: muscle relaxation and breathing; mental focusing; and other deepening techniques. I would suggest that you use these in sequence for each one serves a particular function. When used in conjunction with each other, they will enable you to readily experience a sense of deep mental relaxation.

One point that I should like to emphasise is the need for you to apply all of these in an *effortless* way. From early childhood we are exhorted to *try* hard in everything that we do, the implication being that if we work hard at something, we will always succeed. This is appropriate enough in everyday life, but it is an approach which is counter-productive if you wish to relax your mind. A passive attitude—one of just letting things happen—is the one most likely to take you into a state of mental calmness and detachment.

Muscle relaxation and breathing

Many people expect to be 'out to it' when in hypnosis or self-hypnosis and are thus surprised to find that the prevailing feeling is one of intense relaxation. This is often accompanied by other pleasant sensations such as floatiness, heaviness or the feeling that their limbs no longer belong to their body. It is important that you be aware of this fact otherwise you may believe, mistakenly, that you have not achieved self-hypnosis. Apart from the subjective feelings of relaxation that will occur spontaneously as the result of your using a series of procedures that I will describe later, you will find it helpful also to incorporate a technique of gradually relaxing different parts of the body. The reasons for this are twofold. First, it helps you experience a much deeper state of self-hypnosis[15] and second, it gives you time to settle your body before setting out on the more difficult task of quietening your mind.

You will find it helpful to incorporate your breathing into this muscle relaxation process. Not only does this help to distract you from the temptation of *trying* to relax but breathing has an important role in its own right. As Jencks[16] has suggested 'long, slow, deep exhalations bring about relaxation with the accompanying sensations of sinking, widening, opening up, and softening; the feelings of comfort, heaviness, warmth, and moisture; the moods of patience and calmness'. The feelings you can achieve using this technique are best described in the words of an elite sportsman: 'Each time I breathed out, all the tension was being pushed down into the toes and out of my body'.

It is helpful to start with the small muscles around the eyes and face. You will find it easier, at first, to relax small muscles rather than the large muscle groups of, say, the arms or legs. Focus on the face muscles and as you do so, imagine you are breathing away all tension and strain from those muscles with each exhalation. As the jaw muscles relax, feel the face becoming soft and let the lips part easily and naturally. Once the face muscles feel relaxed, then move to those of the forehead and scalp. Breathe away the tension from them. Some people find it helpful to imagine also that the relaxation is spreading outwards from the face in concentric waves just as ripples spread out on the surface of a still pool when the water is disturbed.

You can then move progressively into the shoulders, upper arms, lower arms, hands and fingers; through the upper back and chest, the lower back and abdomen and slowly down through the legs to the toes. Use your breathing out as a means of releasing the strain and tightness from each area. This relaxation process must be unhurried. It takes a little time for muscles to relax and you may find that certain muscle groups, such as in the neck or shoulders, are especially tense and tight and sometimes take a great deal longer to relax.

As you allow the arms, hands, legs and feet to relax, you may notice certain unusual feelings or sensations. Some people experience a sense of tingling whilst others feel as though their limbs no longer belong to them. If these occur, you need not be concerned. They indicate that you are already starting to achieve your desired goal—mental and physical disengagement.

Mental focusing

Now that your body is feeling perfectly relaxed, it is necessary to move on to the next technique, one aimed at helping you to relax and still your mind. This, in my opinion, is the most important of all the induction procedures. Unfortunately, you may also find that it is the most difficult.

I make no apologies for reiterating the importance of mental focusing. It is, without doubt, the *sine qua non* for achieving a state of complete detachment or disengagement from cares, problems, events of the day. If your mind remains uncontrolled and continually gets caught up in intrusive thoughts, it is unlikely you will be able to experience a significant depth of disengagement and thus, self-hypnosis. A technique to gradually bring your wandering mind under control is all-important. The procedure that I suggest bears a close resemblance to those used in meditation and in the induction of the relaxation response.[17] This is not surprising since the central theme in all of these relaxation states is the stilling of the mind.

How to concentrate your attention

By the time you have completed your physical relaxation process, you may feel very comfortable but still be aware that all sorts of thoughts keep popping into your mind unbidden. How do you get rid of these? The first thing to realise is that you cannot empty your mind of these distracting thoughts by *trying* to shut them out. This will only serve to make them even more intrusive. If you have any doubts on this matter, let me give you a simple task. Try *not* to think of the colour blue. I doubt whether you were thinking of the colour blue before I mentioned it, but I feel sure you are now. This indicates that if you try to shut anything out of your mind, it will cause you to dwell upon it still further.

In order for you to gradually empty your mind it is necessary for it to have something else upon which to focus. This is the basis of the mantra used in meditation. You will find that a monosyllabic word such as 'calm' or 'peace' will be an effective focusing aid. Some people ask whether 'relax' would be a satisfactory word to use. In my opinion, the word itself is unimportant as long as you feel comfortable in using it. My only reservation about the use of 'relax' is that it may engender, once again, an effortful, as opposed to an effortless, approach.

You will find that it helps you to achieve rhythm if you think of, say, 'calm' each time you exhale. At first, it is almost certain that you will find competing thoughts constantly entering your mind. Just accept the inevitability of this occuring and, when it does, re-focus your mind on your centring word. Let these thoughts pass through the mind like visitors—as though they are flowing in through one ear and out the other. You will probably find that such intrusions continue for a while, but eventually the influence of your focusing word will become apparent and other thoughts will gradually recede further and further into the background. Be prepared to spend at least five minutes on this process. Through constant practice, you will find that you are not only able to achieve a still mind, but are able to maintain it for as long as you wish. A variation of this technique, suggested by one of my patients, may help you centre your attention more easily. Each time you think of your focusing word (for example, 'calm'), imagine you are dropping a pebble into a still pool and watch the ripples spread slowly outwards in concentric circles. The main thing is not to become discouraged by your erratic and, at times, perverse unconscious. Some days it will be easier to control than others. In line with this, the depth or intensity of self-hypnosis will appear greater. But be reassured that no matter what degree of depth of self-hypnosis you experience, it will still be of considerable benefit to you.

Other deepening procedures

Once you have brought your mind under control it will be possible to achieve a greater depth of mental relaxation through the use of any one of a number of techniques. Most incorporate mental imagery; some the use of counting. I will describe below a number of techniques and suggest that you select the one that you find suits you best. This may entail trying out a new one from time to time until you feel comfortable and competent with one of them.

A counting procedure

In using this, you count silently from one to twenty. Synchronise the counting of each number with your exhalation. By the time you reach this stage of your induction, you will notice how slow and shallow your breathing has become. As you count, think of each number as being like a stepping stone, taking your mind further and further into a disengaged state. By the time you reach twenty, you will feel a considerable depth of relaxation.

Imagery techniques

There is an unlimited number of ways of deepening self-hypnosis using visualisation or mental imagery techniques. The ones that I will describe are only intended as guidelines: many people use their own ingenuity to develop individual imaginal techniques. You can be quite eclectic in the manner in which you use your imagination to deepen self-hypnosis.

People vary greatly in the ways that they can imagine. Some are extremely imaginative, this characteristic occurring more frequently in those of an artistic bent and also in elite sportspeople. Such people use imaginative techniques in hypnosis and self-hypnosis with ease.

At the other end of the spectrum are those who are unable to form mental pictures. If you have difficulty imagining things, accept that this is not one of your strengths and use another deepening procedure such as counting.

The descending-steps method As you rest back in self-hypnosis, visualise yourself standing at the top of twenty steps or stairs. Imagine that these steps lead to a very tranquil scene—one in which you can feel totally relaxed and at peace. The imagery of the steps and the scene may be based on some experience you recall from the past. On the other hand, it may be one that your mind constructs as being pleasant, one that it would like to escape to in moments of tension and anxiety. While it is best to let your imagination unfold the mental picture in its own way, this is not to say that you cannot change the setting from one session to the next. Let it all happen in an effortless way.

Having visualised the steps and scene below, picture yourself descending each step quite slowly. You will probably find it helpful to synchronise the descent of each step with each breath out. As you descend each step, count silently from one until the count of twenty at the bottom. Think of each step as being a level of relaxation so that you go deeper into self-hypnosis as you descend. You may wish to stop from time to time and take in the view. Let the whole process happen as naturally and in as an unstructured way as possible.

Once you have arrived at the bottom of the steps, feel free to go into your selected scene. You can rest in that imagined scene for as long as you wish and experience a complete sense of peace and mental detachment.

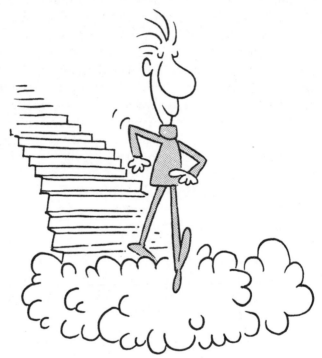

Picture yourself descending to a tranquil scene

The blackboard technique   Whatever imaginal techniques you use to induce self-hypnosis, they all serve to intensify a state of involvement or absorption, and help you to further narrow your attention. One such technique devised by Stanton[18] utilises the visualisation of a blackboard or whiteboard.

As you picture the blackboard in your mind's eye, imagine that written on it are the numbers one to twenty. Once you have that image firmly fixed, you picture each number being erased and, as you do so, think of the words 'let go'. Again, synchronise the words with your exhalation phase as if you are breathing out the words. You will feel a sense of letting go of tension, worries and intrusions with each number you erase.

A variation of the mental blackboard technique was suggested by a patient, who found that rubbing out numbers involved him in too much mental effort. (This emphasises the importance of your feeling free to modify any procedure so that it suits *you*, rather than trying to follow, to the letter, the ones I suggest.) He preferred to see each number slowly fading away like a scene dissolving on a movie screen, and then being gradually replaced by the next number. As each number dissolved away, he thought of the words 'let go' and felt an increasing sense of letting go of tension and concerns as he did so.

Many people prefer the blackboard technique because of the freedom it gives them in controlling the rate at which they 'let go' of anxious thoughts and tension. Furthermore, I have noticed that even those who have a low imaginative capacity are able to visualise a blackboard. A possible explanation for this is the early conditioning we all have as schoolchildren.

Your mental lift   In the deepening techniques described so far, there has been a finite point at which they stopped, for example, at the count of twenty. Most people are content to experience whatever intensity of self-hypnosis that these techniques bring them. Others have indicated to me that they feel restricted by these and would like to be able to take themselves to an even greater depth. For such people (who invariably possess a high imaginative capacity) there is the mental lift procedure.

You imagine yourself seated in a most comfortable lounge chair which is situated in your own mental lift. This lift is unlike any you have ever seen because it is spacious and you are surrounded by pleasant things—your own furniture, flowers, paintings. As you rest back in your chair, you have at your fingertips a mechanism with which you can control the descent and ascent of the lift. On a small screen in front of you are numbers indicating the levels of relaxation that you can achieve in your mental lift.

When you are ready to take yourself deeper into self-hypnosis, you start the lift, and as it passes through each level you see the number light up on the screen. You will probably notice how slowly the lift moves—everything is unhurried and free from tension. There is no limit to the depth of relaxation you can achieve. The more levels you pass through, the deeper your state of disengagement.

When you reach the level which seems appropriate for you, you stop the lift and as the doors open, step out into a scene of peace. Some visualise an outdoor scene such as an exotic garden; others prefer to step into a cool, quiet beautifully furnished room. Once in that scene, you can rest and enjoy it for as long as you wish.

Two points emerge from the use of this technique. First, you should not predetermine the level of relaxation you wish to experience but simply allow your mind to achieve the depth in which you feel comfortable on that particular occasion. Second, you should allow the scene you go into to develop spontaneously. Many find that this more unstructured approach leads to a sense of effortlessness, a condition which, as I have already emphasised, is always to be encouraged if you wish to achieve an optimal level of mental disengagement.

How do I come out of it?

At this stage, you are possibly having the same thought as do many of my patients: 'Now that I can take myself into self-hypnosis, how can I bring myself out of it?' As stated earlier, this presents no particular difficulty. You could, for instance, simply open your eyes when you are ready to do so, but it is advisable to use a cue to bring it to a close and to terminate it gradually. This will ensure that you have no 'hangover' effects such as drowsiness or unsteadiness when you stand up.

Before you bring your self-hypnosis to a close, it is advisable for you to reverse your deepening procedure. Thus, if you have descended twenty steps, imagine coming back up these as you count from twenty back to one. Or, if you have used your mental lift, bring it back gently to its starting level. A further method of 'counteracting' the deepening effects is to give yourself the suggestion 'My mind is becoming peacefully blank; all images are fading away'. This reversal process is to ensure that you do not come out of self-hypnosis with the feeling that, somehow, you are still partially in your relaxing, peaceful scene. In most cases, this is unlikely to happen, but if you are highly hypnotisable it is possible that your disengaged feelings will persist for a while unless you have taken the trouble to reverse them.

As a way of terminating self-hypnosis, I recommend counting silently from five back to one and allowing the eyes to open at 'one'. If you still feel unduly drowsy or disorientated, it helps to make a few energetic movements such as stretching and bending your arms.

Be assured that there is no danger of you being 'left' in self-hypnosis, unable to move and unable to bring yourself out of it. The worst that can happen is that you allow your deep state of relaxation to drift into a normal sleep state. This is more likely to occur when you are tired, and if it does happen, you will waken from it feeling quite refreshed after a short while.

CHAPTER FOUR

SELF-HYPNOSIS AS A THERAPY

Now that you have learned how you can achieve a still and relaxed mind, it is necessary to look at the ways in which you can use this state to gain control over stress-related problems. This is, after all, the reason for using it. As pleasant as a state of relaxation is, it will not provide you with the coping skills necessary for dealing with anxiety problems. The game plan, so to speak, is to help you gradually change those negative behaviours that bother you and replace them with more positive responses. This is the therapeutic phase of the self-hypnosis program.

Having realistic expectations

Before you embark on the use of self-hypnosis, there are two aspects that should be emphasised. The first concerns the need to use self-hypnosis on a regular basis so that it becomes integrated into your lifestyle. This will ensure that you achieve a progressive improvement in the management of your problems, and also prevents a relapse of the symptoms. The second centres on the importance of having realistic expectations concerning your rate of improvement.

Unfortunately, with regard to health, we all tend to be impatient and expect improvement to occur in the shortest possible time. Some people have more unrealistic expectations than others and become discouraged if anticipated changes do not happen in the first few weeks. This leads to them abandoning the use of self-hypnosis, viewing it as being of little benefit to them. I like to illustrate the need for patience and continuing use of the procedure by drawing two graphs. The first depicts the belief held by some people that significant changes will occur once the treatment has started. They anticipate that, after a short while, their symptoms will drop to low levels and remain that way, as shown on the graph below.

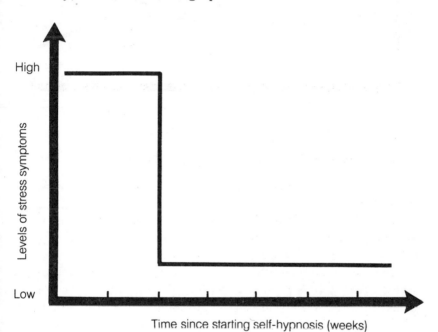

Time since starting self-hypnosis (weeks)

It must be emphasised that this is quite unrealistic. Usually, improvement tends to be a gradual process and may be interspersed with occasions when your symptoms recur. At other times, your condition may remain unchanged in spite of your continuing use of self-hypnosis.[11]Many become demoralised when confronted by these events. What you have to realise is that producing changes in any behaviour requires time *and* effort on your part. You should anticipate setbacks or plateaus (as depicted in the graph), but they will be temporary in nature.

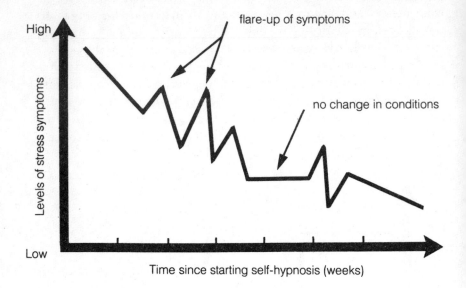

Your therapeutic approach

There are three ways you can capitalise on your relaxed, sensitive state of mind:
—by giving yourself positive suggestions or affirmations;
—through the use of problem solving; and
—by utilising self-hypnotic imagery.

Each of these procedures can produce significant changes within you, and in your behaviours. You may not find it necessary to call upon all three approaches each time you enter self-hypnosis, but they are all available for you to use if you feel the need.

THE VALUE OF POSITIVE SELF-SUGGESTIONS

Over the years, there have been many schools of 'positive thinking'. One of the earliest was that of Coué in 1922. Suggestions that he presented to patients included one that is familiar to many: 'Tous les jours, à tous points de vue, je vais de mieux en mieux,' ('Day by day, in every way, I'm getting better and better'). Coué intended that patients repeat this phrase to themselves each day to produce a more positive attitude towards themselves and the way that they felt. However, the use of such a psychological litany has been criticised by some as being too general to help a person develop ways of coping with specific problems.

While this criticism may be justified, it is certainly true that the things we say to ourselves each day influence the way we feel and respond. We all tend to talk to ourselves; usually this is silent, but occasionally we may even talk out loud. Sometimes this 'inner conversation', as some psychologists call it (I prefer 'self-talk'), takes place outside our conscious awareness. On other occasions we realise that we are giving ourselves negative suggestions but have no means at our disposal to combat them.

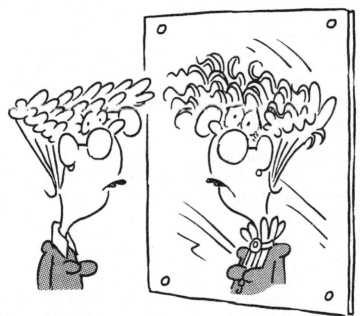

Our 'self-talk' can influence the way we feel and respond

How negative thoughts affect you

How often have you internally verbalised the following types of thoughts when faced by some difficulty? 'I hope that I can manage to do this all right. It would be awful if I don't succeed. What would [specifying the person or people] think of me if I don't do it properly? I don't feel too confident about tackling this. Perhaps it's because I don't feel up-to-the-mark today. If I fail, that is going to make me feel terrible.'

Negative thoughts such as these, particularly if they are reinforced over many occasions, inevitably lead you into negative patterns of behaviour. You feel tense and anxious, lose confidence in your ability to carry out tasks and, because you fear that you will not please others, your self-esteem is undermined. Just as negative thoughts lead to negative feelings so, too, do positive, realistic thoughts create a sense of buoyancy, positive expectation and a sense of well-being.

It would seem reasonable to argue that, if it is so easy to make ourselves feel better, react ideally in various situations and generally cope by simply giving ourselves positive thoughts, why don't more people do it? Unfortunately, as I have already indicated, much of our thinking occurs at an unconscious level. We may not be aware that we are constantly 'programming' negative thoughts into our mind. While these thoughts are often subtle in nature (for example, 'I've never been much good at maths,' or 'I'm hopeless at serving when I play tennis'), they can still have a damaging effect on our responses and behaviours.

An inclination towards negative patterns of thinking is often associated with feelings of stress or depression. The anxious or depressed person is far more inclined to ruminate on, and worry about things that have happened in the past and might happen in the future. The tendency to dwell on the past and the effect that it has had (what I term the 'if only' syndrome) can so often preoccupy people that they lose sight of the importance of recognising the good things in themselves and their lives *in the present*. We have had times when we have been troubled by thoughts such as 'If only I had made a different decision, I would not be in the position I am today'. Sometimes it does help to reflect on certain happenings in the past, but *only* if it can be seen as a positive step towards helping you cope more effectively with the here-and-now.

The 'what if' syndrome is also prevalent in people who are stressed. Invariably, this is associated with low self-esteem, and is characterised by thought processes such as: 'I would like to take a year off work and do that special course. I know that I will benefit from it. But *what if* I don't succeed? Wouldn't that be awful. I will have wasted a year and everyone will think badly of me.'

When we are calm and rational most of us realise that there is little to be gained by constantly reviewing unpleasant past happenings, or negatively anticipating future events. But in an anxious state such thoughts are profoundly intrusive, serving to intensify our stress still further.

The role of positive thinking

How you go about reversing these negative patterns of thought will depend upon, first, being able to identify that you do tend to think in this way. This may not be as easy task, especially if you are experiencing chronic stress problems or if you have established a long-standing habit of approaching things in your life in a negative way.

Once you have recognised that you are constantly being trapped in negative thoughts you will be well on the way to putting the situation to rights. Behavioural psychologists have been interested for many years in studying the effects of self-statements on a person's responses or behaviours. This is known as cognitive psychology. Several forms of therapy have arisen from these studies, rational-emotive therapy (RET)[19] and stress-innoculation training[20] being among the better known. All such therapies teach patients to recognise the presence and understand the role of negative self-statements and train them in coping techniques.

Clearly, the things you say to yourself, whether negative or positive, will have a deep and lasting effect on the way you behave. If you can find a way of restructuring your negative thoughts through the use of positive self-suggestion, then this will help considerably in reducing your stress and anxiety levels.

Self-hypnosis provides an ideal medium in which to do this. In the state of relaxation and disengagement that characterises hypnosis and self-hypnosis, the mind is much more responsive to suggestions. Patients who have experienced the induction of hypnosis by someone else are often concerned that the suggestions that they give to themselves in self-hypnosis may not be as effective as those given in hypnosis. Their concerns are groundless. As Salter states, 'It doesn't make any difference *who* gives you the suggestions . . .they may come from within or without. As long as you cooperate, with me or with yourself, the suggestions work'.[21]

The correct framing of suggestions

Initially you might be uncertain as to what sort of suggestions you are to give yourself once you have induced self-hypnosis. This is seldom a problem for a therapist using hypnosis, for he or she is in the comfortable position of not only understanding the areas requiring treatment, but also in having the expertise to provide the appropriate suggestion.

Obviously, the suggestions that you give to yourself are determined by the nature of your problem, but there are certain guidelines which may help. Suggestions should be as brief as possible, relevant to your problem and *always* structured in a positive way. If you use such negative self-suggestions as 'I am not going to let it worry me,' or 'I am not going to let the pain bother me,' it will cause your mind to focus on the very things you are trying to change.

Your work diary

Writing positive suggestions that you can give yourself in a notebook will enable you to correctly frame and memorise them, so that you can use them in self-hypnosis in an effortless way. As you become familiar with them, you will have less need to refer to your book.

It is important to keep a work diary if you are to gain the most out of self-therapy. It is intended as a personal record and, as you will see later, it will help you work through problems. It will also provide a yardstick with which you can gauge your progress. It is all too easy to forget how badly you coped in the past. If you can compare past behaviour with present it will motivate you to continue using self-hypnosis.

The nature of suggestions

Suggestions can be broadly divided into two categories: those that are non-specific which will help you establish better self-confidence and self-esteem, and those that are tailored to help you cope with a specific problem.

Whether you use the first or second person, i.e. 'I am going to . . .' or 'You are going to . . .' does not seem to be significant. It has been my experience that most people prefer to give suggestions in the first person. Needless to say, all suggestions are presented silently, as though you are talking to yourself.

General coping suggestions

General coping suggestions (some call them ego-strengthening suggestions[22]) are useful as a means of helping rebuild your self-confidence and self-esteem, and allaying anxiety. Structured in such a way that they are readily accepted by the mind as factual, it is more effective if you express them in your own phraseology rather than follow someone else's formula.

The following suggestions are provided merely as guidelines:

'Now that I am in this very relaxed
state . . .my mind feels so sensitive . . .and
the suggestions I give to myself . . .are going to
help me, each day, achieve the things I want
to achieve.'

'The feelings of relaxation that I have
now . . .are going to carry through into every
part of my day.'

'I will become much more aware of feelings of
relaxation . . .coming into the whole of my
body—into every cell . . .every
organ . . .every muscle . . .so that, little by
little . . .I am going to experience a greater
sense of physical wellbeing and ease.'

'Not only will I become more relaxed in my body . . .I will enjoy a greater sense of tranquillity and peace in my mind. My mind will feel so much clearer . . .and no matter what problems arise in daily life . . .I will feel that I can keep them in perspective . . .without magnifying or distorting them in any way.'

'As these pleasant feelings of relaxation gradually develop within me . . .I am going to experience a sense of increasing confidence and self-assurance . . .in all types of situations and in all types of company.'

'I will notice too . . .that I am more able to recognise the good things in myself . . .my own special attributes . . .my own strengths. I am going to feel so comfortable . . .about focusing in on these.'

'Because of this, my respect for myself . . .for my body . . .for my health is going to continue to grow . . .and I will feel an increasing desire to protect my body against the harmful effects of constant stress . . .by becoming more relaxed.'

'With these greater feelings of relaxation in my mind . . .in my body . . .I will realise, more and more . . .that I can respond . . .in quite a different way . . .from in the past. I can become a much stronger person than I was before . . .and be able to cope with things . . .that would have upset me previously.'

The purpose of each self-suggestion should be to promote positive change within you and, as you will notice, the central theme is that of relaxation.

Recognising the problem

The second type of suggestion—specific coping suggestions—are those that you can give yourself to deal with specific problem areas in your life. The essential first step, however, is for you to be able to recognise the nature of what is bothering you. Generally this may not prove a difficulty, but you might find there are occasions when it is quite hard to identify why you are unable to cope satisfactorily with a particular situation, person or event, or why you react inappropriately to things that happen in your life. This state of mental confusion often stems from stress. Self-hypnosis helps to quieten the mind so that you can gain a better insight into the things that bother you.

One way that people commonly attempt to deal with problems is through denial. Trying to convince yourself that a problem is not really there, and hoping that it will go away if you do not think about it, is unrealistic and prevents you developing suitable coping skills. Recognising and confronting the problem is the platform on which you build your self-management and self-control skills.

It is not until you start to look constructively at the problem areas in your life and at the way in which you react to them that you realise how frequently you approach them in a negative way. Sometimes this entails your taking steps to actively avoid the issue that bothers you. A variation of this avoidance strategy may arise from your belief that you cannot succeed in doing a particular thing and therefore it is not worthwhile trying in the first instance. These negative self-statements and beliefs can only lead to negative patterns of behaviour. You become more stressed, your self-esteem and self-confidence are further undermined, and so you approach similar situations in the future with ever decreasing expectations of success. You are now well on the way to establishing a vicious cycle: stress ⟶ negative patterns of thinking ⟶ increased stress. With each experience, you sensitise yourself still further to respond negatively. It is little wonder that people frequently reach a point where they feel unable to cope with even the smallest amount of stress in their lives.

Breaking the negative thought cycle

If you are to break the vicious cycle that you have established (often over a long period of time), it will become necessary to 'reprogram' your mind with a new set of suggestions. This plan of attack on your stress starts with a firm decision to recognise every occasion in your daily life when you dwell on negative self-talk, and then to set about replacing such episodes with positive, coping suggestions. An allegory that I like to use with my patients may give you an illustration of what I mean.

Let us imagine that you are bushwalking or tramping and you arrive at the base of a mountain. As you gaze at the steepness of the slope and the severity of the terrain, two possible internal monologues can take place. The negative one would go something like this:

> '*Well, that mountain certainly looks daunting. It would be nice to get to the top. I expect the views would be magnificent. But I feel quite tired and the day is hot. I might even injure myself or get lost on the way up. It's probably best that I don't start on it—it would be awful to get only part of the way up and then have to turn round. That would take up so much time and energy, and I don't think I can be bothered in any case.*'

Contrast this with one which promotes positive, coping suggestions:

> *That mountain looks quite steep and I expect that the climb will be difficult at times [realistic expectations]. I should like to get to the top—not only will this make me feel that I have achieved something but the views will be spectacular. It will make me feel good in future to be able to look at the mountain and know that I have conquered it [reinforcing positive self-statements]. I'm going to climb it slowly, at my own pace. When I feel tired, I*

will stop and rest. I may have a drink and take in the view. By doing it in this way, I will eventually get to the top and enjoy the views and the sense of freedom that it brings [coping suggestions].

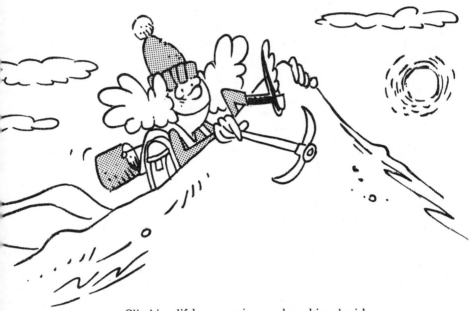

Climbing life's mountains can be achieved with positive self-talk

Life is full of such mountains for all of us. Whether we experience success and a sense of achievement is so often governed by the things we say to ourselves. It becomes much easier to formulate positive self-suggestions if we are in a relaxed frame of mind, and this is where self-hypnosis can be so beneficial.

The value of a relaxation cue mechanism

Giving yourself positive thoughts in self-hypnosis will, in time, produce positive feelings within you. You may find it extremely helpful to be able to reinforce these effects in daily life through the use of a cue mechanism. This cue is designed to act as a mental 'bell ringer', reminding you to relax and respond in a particular way.

The one I recommend is to think of the word 'calm' as you breathe out, and to do so for fifteen to twenty seconds at a time. This will be equivalent to four to five breaths. If you repeat this mini-relaxation twenty to thirty times each day in a variety of situations, it will become so powerful and ingrained that your mind can call upon it whenever you feel your stress levels rising.

In a sense, it is not unlike an airconditioning unit which has been set on automatic function. If the room temperature rises, this causes the thermostat to switch on the air cooler, which brings conditions back to a level where you feel comfortable. A relaxation cue which has become conditioned by regular reinforcement will do much the same thing by bringing your stress down to a state where you feel at ease again.

HOW TO EMPLOY SPECIFIC COPING SUGGESTIONS

As in the case of general coping suggestions, you may find it helpful to write down in your work diary the types of self-statements that you are going to implement. This will give you the opportunity to study and memorise them before you embark on self-therapy, and will enable you to recognise any negative self-talk that might inadvertently have crept in (for example, 'I am *not* going to get upset by . . .' or 'I am going to try and *not* let it worry me').

Clearly, because of the wide variety of difficulties that confront people, it is possible to provide examples of only a few specific coping suggestions. I have chosen obesity as a model because it is a problem which confronts a great many people, and is often associated with 'wrong thinking'.

The control of obesity

Obesity in one of the major health concerns in the Western world and because of people's concerns over the effect that excessive weight has on their health and wellbeing, a huge industry has been spawned to encourage people to shed excess kilograms. Rarely a week passes without some new diet being promoted. It stands to reason that if any one diet was markedly effective, we would not continually be hearing of new ones.

Perhaps the principal reason why so many diets are unsuccessful is that they fail to confront the underlying psychological mechanisms that initially precipitate a person's poor eating habits. Unless factors such as stress and low self-esteem are dealt with, any attempts at satisfactory weight loss are going to prove ineffectual in the long term.

The effect of negative self-talk

What you say to yourself may have a most damaging effect on your attempt to establish a sound eating pattern that will be acceptable, cause you to lose weight gradually and enable you to maintain your weight at its optimal level. People tend to reinforce bad eating behaviours by constantly using a great deal of negative self-talk. There are many examples of negative inner speech that I could draw on, but the following should be sufficient to give you an insight into how damaging these can be.

I have tried to lose weight many times before, but it only lasts for a short while and then goes up again.

I can't resist eating sweet things. I have no willpower—I can't seem to stop myself.

I would eat the right things but it's no use cooking them because the children won't like them.

Once I start eating, I can't seem to stop until I feel full.

Replacing the bad thoughts

Once you have recognised that these types of negative thoughts are creeping into your mind, you are well on the way to changing them for more desirable coping suggestions given in self-hypnosis:

> *I am going to learn to relax a little more each day . . .and as I do so, I will notice how much more confident I become in my approach to eating. I will find it easier to plan my meals . . .the food that I eat . . .just changing my eating in small ways at first . . .until my new pattern of eating becomes a habit.*

> *Instead of worrying about willpower . . .I am going to feel an ever-increasing unconscious need within me to gradually control what I eat . . .how much I eat.*

> *I am going to enjoy eating small helpings of vegetables . . .fruit . . .fish . . .poultry . . .chewing each mouthful slowly . . .so that I can savour it for as long as possible. When I leave the dining table . . .I will feel stimulated by the thought . . .that I was content to eat a small helping. Eating too much . . .is damaging to my body. My body is important to me . . .and because I now feel a greater respect for my body . . .I want to protect it . . .from the harmful effects of being overweight.*

The goal in using these specific coping suggestions is to *gradually* modify your behaviours and attitudes. Weight loss must, of necessity, be gradual, so be patient. Set goals but not unrealistic ones. See the need to change your mental approach as being the springboard for your weight loss. Appropriate suggestions in self-hypnosis will help you achieve those goals.

PROBLEMS AND HOW TO RESOLVE THEM

The second way in which you gainfully apply self-hypnosis is the resolution of problems. How often have you been confronted by concerns which, at the time, appeared almost impossible to resolve? Sometimes these can arise from a deep-seated anxiety which interferes with your ability to put troubling situations into perspective and thus be able to resolve them in a clear, logical fashion. On other occasions your appropriate responses are influenced by the way that you dealt with similar problems in the past. If, for instance, you coped poorly with a previous situation then, to some extent, you will have been unconsciously sensitised into negatively anticipating that the same thing will happen again. It follows, therefore, that if you are to learn how to deal more effectively with your problems, you have to be prepared to change your approach in some way.

Piecing together your mental jigsaw puzzle

Without question, the mental relaxation which stems from using self-hypnosis will go a long way towards helping you look at difficulties more clearly. It will allow you to put things into their true perspective. But this may not be sufficient, in itself, to fit all the pieces of the mind's jigsaw puzzle back in place.

You may need some extra techniques in order to do this, and self-hypnosis can provide you with an ideal environment for confronting and learning new ways of resolving problems that may be bothering you. In this state of mental and physical relaxation, you will have the opportunity to look at your concerns in as much or as little detail as you wish. In other words you do not *have* to face up to the whole problem area all at once if you feel uncomfortable in doing so. Instead, you can let it unfold gradually, over a number of sessions.

You may wonder about the wisdom of confronting the things that bother you. Your thoughts may go something like this: 'It's all very well suggesting that I look at my problems and try and resolve them in a new way. But I have already spent a considerable part of my life dwelling on them and that hasn't done much for me except make them worse on occasions. It appears that the more I think about them, the worse they become. Why should your technique make things any easier?' This argument, although understandable, is flawed. For one thing, I am asking you to confront the problem in a relaxed, peaceful state of mind instead of worrying about it in a highly stressed state.

In self-hypnosis you can study a problem in your life without being constantly bombarded by self-doubts and feelings of guilt or self-recrimination. There is a great deal of difference between unhelpful worry and constructive thinking and planning. Previously you faced your worries without your having any effective psychological means of dealing with them. Now you can confront them safe in the knowledge that you have much sounder coping skills. The feeling you get from using self-hypnosis in this way is best described in the words of one of my patients: 'I used to feel that I was completely unarmed in trying to deal with all the problems in my life. Now I feel as though I have a strong weapon, which guards me all the time.'

Problem-solving with your work diary

Earlier in this chapter, I suggested that you establish a work diary. You will find that this will be of considerable help in your problem-solving, too, for by writing down the problem situation as you experience it, it will enable you to view it in a much more objective way—to stand back from it, as it were.

Some people find it hard to set out their problems on paper. They are embarrassed by having to reveal to themselves the things that bother them, feeling as if they are baring their soul. One of the best ways of getting around this is to write out your problems as if you are telling someone about them. Write down the things that trouble you, how you feel about them and even some of the possible ways of dealing with them. You may be surprised to find that writing out the problem is often sufficient to give you a good insight into how you can best resolve it. If setting it out on paper fails to resolve the problem, however, you should not be discouraged. You are now in a position to study it, free from other outside concerns, in self-hypnosis.

There are a number of ways that this can be carried out. Some incorporate the use of imagery procedures, and these will be dealt with later in this chapter. Others involve thinking of the problem, in self-hypnosis, in a detached fashion. This is not unlike watching a video replay of various past situations in your life where the problem has affected you. Re-experiencing those situations, how you reacted and what your thoughts were, will often give a clearer insight of how the problem is affecting you. Once you are aware of your negative reactions to the problem, you will have the opportunity to visualise yourself coping with that same situation in a satisfactory way, i.e. replacing negative responses with positive ones.

Once you have analysed the problem in self-hypnosis, you may find it helpful to review the possible ways of resolving it—ones that you have written in your work diary. Being able to look at each of these in a relaxed state enables you to select one as the most appropriate way of dealing with your concern. Alternatively, you may reach the conclusion that you are worrying about something which lies outside your control. If this is the case, you should suggest to yourself that you are going to put that worry on a 'special shelf' in your mind which is solely reserved for things you cannot influence. Acknowledging that you are worrying unnecessarily, and then giving yourself permission to put that concern onto a special 'worries shelf' will help you release the problem.

MENTAL IMAGERY IN SELF-HYPNOSIS

Mental imagery is a concept that is familiar to most of us. After all, who has not spent some part of their life daydreaming? Fantasy tends to be more involving in childhood: one has only to watch children at play in order to gain an insight into the way in which the human mind can induce intense fantasies. Children seem to have the capacity to 'lose themselves' in an imagined role to the extent that it becomes reality to them. As we get older, this imaginative capacity usually diminishes, but most of us retain some ability to fantasise.

Your imaginative ability

The degree to which we can experience imagery varies considerably from person to person, some people having an immense capacity for imaginative involvement.[12]

A person's imaginative capacity is a personality characteristic. Some of us, when asked to visualise a situation, can do so with such intensity that we feel as though we are actually experiencing it. Others are able to imagine but with far less intensity, whilst there are those who have great difficulty in picturing anything in their mind's eye. Clearly, if you are in the latter group, visualisation techniques in self-hypnosis are not for you. A simple test to determine whether you can use imagery techniques is to close your eyes and try to picture a scene that is familiar to you, such as your garden at home. If you are successful in 'seeing' the various features of your garden, you can feel quite confident is using imaginal procedures in your self-therapy.

Why imagery is effective

Imagery by itself is a most potent tool in many forms of therapy. It has been widely applied in behaviour modification and psychotherapy for many years and when it is linked with self-hypnosis, it becomes even more effective. In the state of mental disengagement that characterises self-hypnosis, there is an even greater opportunity for involvement in imagery. Imagined scenes become more intense, to such an extent that highly hypnotisable people are often able to experience all the sensations associated with the situation. If they visualise a garden scene, for example, they smell the fragrance of flowers, feel the gentle breeze, hear the sounds of birds and insects just as though they were there in real life. It is this capacity for imaginative experiences that renders self-hypnotic imagery so valuable. But it should not be thought that these beneficial effects are solely restricted to the more highly hypnotisable subjects. Even in the absence of these intense experiences, imagery still enables you to *make mental contact with situations* whilst in a state of complete relaxation, so that you can gain insight into and modify the things in your behaviour that you wish to change.

Techniques of self-hypnotic imagery

There are a great many ways in which you can use your powers of imagination in self-hypnosis. It is helpful to review these under the following headings:

—to attain a state of inner quiet;
—as a means of confronting and gaining insight into a problem;
—for the removal of a problem or symptom;
—as a way of desensitising yourself from a feared situation; and
—imagery rehearsal.

You may find that you need to incorporate several of these approaches into your self-treatment program at any one time.

Your inner mental place

Once you have attained your optimal depth of relaxation using the techniques described in Chapter 3, you may wish to enjoy, for a while, a state of quietness of mind, but you will quickly become aware that unless you involve your mind in some procedure, intrusive thoughts ('mental noise' as some people describe it) soon reappear. To achieve this state of inner peace you can use your own inner mental place.[23,24]

I am walking slowly . . .along a
beautiful . . .peaceful corridor of my mind.
[You can imagine anything you wish in this
corridor. Some people like to visualise an
exotic scene such as a miniaturised Hall of
Mirrors from the Palace of Versailles. Others,
a more simple image of palm trees and gardens
or fine paintings on the walls.] This corridor
is taking me . . .into my own . . .inner mental
place. I notice an ornate door . . .and as I
open it . . .find myself in a beautiful
scene . . .one of
peace . . .tranquillity . . .where
nothing . . .nor any one . . .can damage or
harm me. As I close the door behind me . . .I
feel as though I am shutting out . . .all
negative thoughts . . .concerns . . .worries. I
am in a state of complete peace . . .and am
going to enjoy . . .exploring this special place
in my mind.

This special place in your mind can also be used to confront and explore a problem that troubles you. It may be one that you have written down in your work diary beforehand. Your inner sanctuary, where your mind is unencumbered by tensions and concerns, provides an ideal situation for looking at your difficulties in a clear, logical way. With the insight that this process provides, you will be able to develop more effective coping skills. Sometimes you will find that you are able to solve the problem quite spontaneously in self-hypnosis. On other occasions the best way of dealing with the problem may come to you at a later time, as though the mind has become disentangled from the web of anxiety. Yet again, you may realise that the problem lies outside your control and nothing you do can influence it. Once you are aware of this, you will find it much easier to place it on a special 'shelf' in your mind— one that is reserved for problems *you* cannot control. This is reinforced by giving yourself the suggestion that you are going to direct your mental efforts towards things in your life that you *can* influence in a constructive way.

You may prefer to use a variation of this technique involving a mental chute to get rid of the things that bother you.[25]

As I walk slowly . . .along a beautiful
corridor of my mind . . .I come to a
door . . .which leads to my inner mental
place. But before I go through that door . . .I
am going to spend a while . . .thinking of some
of the things that bother me . . .that interfere
with my quality of life. [These may be
particular problems or symptoms.] And as I
think about each one . . .I am going to drop it
down a mental chute. [This is not unlike a
laundry chute and you will find it beside the
door that leads to your special place.] As I
dwell upon each difficulty . . .and drop it
down my mental chute . . .I will be able to let
go of it . . .feel that it no longer bothers me.
Now that I have released . . .all the problems
that bother me . . .I can go through the

door . . .into my own inner mental place. A
place of peace and tranquillity . . .

Obviously, this technique enables you to review certain
problems and consider whether you are ready to let go of them.
As with all imagery techniques, you should bring yourself out
of the scene, as it were, by returning through the door and
retracing your steps up the mind's corridor before you terminate
self-hypnosis.

Your mind's double screen

Another imaginal technique, which allows you to confront and
cope with your problems, is the double screen.[14]

Now that I am in a relaxed . . . peaceful . . .
state . . .I see myself resting back . . .in a
very comfortable chair. I can see two large
screens . . .like cinema screens . . .side by
side. The left-hand one . . .is my problem
screen. I can project onto it . . .any problem
that bothers me . . .study it . . .see how I
usually react to it.
I would like to get rid of that problem . . .so I
will switch on the right-hand one . . .my
resolution screen. It will help me . . .
understand a better way . . .of dealing with
my difficulties. I will look at all the possible
ways . . .of reacting better to them. One of
these . . .is going to help me . . .respond just
as I would like.

How to let go of your problems

When you are aware of the things that trouble you (either
thoughts or symptoms) you may wish to use an imaginal
technique that will help you let go of them. The first of these
is the floating leaf procedure:[26]

I can imagine myself . . .sitting in the shade
of a tree . . .on a soft . . .grassy bank of a
stream . . .gazing at the crystal clear

*water . . .trickling gently over the smooth
pebbles and stones. The sounds of the running
water . . .are so soothing . . .I feel at peace in
my scene.*

*A gentle breeze is rustling the leaves of the tree.
One drifts slowly to the ground beside me. As I
pick it up . . .I think of how good it would
be . . .to put my problem . . .on that
leaf . . .and let go of it.*

*Now I can place the leaf . . .gently . . .on the
water. . .and release it . . .watching it float
gently away from me. It reminds me . . .of a
tiny ship . . .as it gently . . .bobs this
way . . .and that . . .getting smaller . . .as the
stream carries my problem . . .further . . .and
further from me. It is disappearing . . .taking
my concern . . .right away from my mind. I
don't need . . .to be bothered . . .by that
problem any longer.*

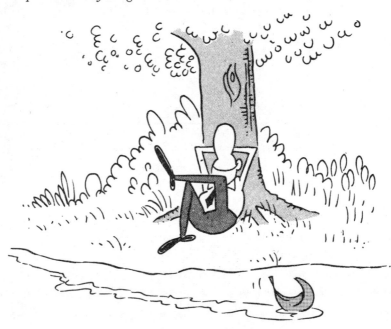

Imagine the problem floating away

You can let go of as many concerns as you wish using this technique. Spend some time thinking of each problem that bothers you before deciding to release it, then let it float away. Just feel a sense of letting go, as though you no longer have need to be troubled by it.

Another imaginal method of releasing problems or concerns is to use the red balloon technique:

I can imagine a large . . .red balloon . . .filled
with helium . . .and a basket is suspended
beneath it. On the ground nearby . . .there is
a small box . . .it is quite empty. I see
myself . . .sitting quietly on the
grass . . .thinking of the symptoms . . .and
difficulties that bother me.
As I think of each one . . .I place it in the
box . . .until I have no more to consider. I
can now place the box in the basket . . .release
the balloon . . .and watch it float high up into
the blue sky . . .getting smaller all the
time . . .until it becomes a tiny red
dot . . .and disappears. I feel a sense of inner
ease . . .at being able to release . . .all my
difficulties.

In all self-hypnotic procedures, you should choose whatever imagery suits you best. One of my patients preferred to visualise herself climbing into the basket with her boxful of problems and, as the balloon rose high into the air, she would drop each one over the side. She felt that she could release her problems more easily using this technique.

Fears and how to deal with them

We have all experienced fears. In childhood, we are inclined to be fearful of such things as the dark and animals. As we get older, our fear pattern tends to change. Many of the things that we fear appear in situations where there is a threat to our well-being or survival. They include confinement in a small space, snakes, insects and heights. These fears are recognised as having an evolutionary basis. In the dim and distant past, our forebears had the same fears: if they had not, many would have perished from such things as poisonous bites or falls from a great height.

It is not this type of fear that concerns us. We accept that if we tried to jump across a chasm and missed our footing then this would almost certainly result in severe injury or death. What bothers most people are the inappropriate fears—those fears we know to be irrational but yet cannot overcome.

Some of these fears can arise as the result of some earlier trauma (for example, a person bitten by a dog may be quite fearful of all dogs thereafter). Others occur without any apparent prior conditioning—they have a certain 'out of the blue' quality about them. It is this type of fear which is so prevalent and which needs treatment.

Reducing your fear sensitivity   The most important aspect of treatment of all fears is exposure. This entails getting closer and closer to the feared situation until you become desensitised to it. In other words, you can tolerate it without undue feelings of anxiety and distress. Exposure therapy may be carried out in real-life situations, and this is the favoured technique of many behavioural psychologists.

Another way of approaching the thing that you fear is by using your imagery in hypnosis or self-hypnosis. This will enable you to imagine a scene some distance (either in time or proximity) from the thing you fear. Thus, if you feel fearful about having to give a talk to a group in an afternoon tutorial, you may, at first, picture yourself at home on the morning of the address. Alternatively, if you have a fear of driving across a bridge, your first scene may involve sitting in your car in your driveway.

Initially you may be quite fearful even in the imagined scene far removed from the thing you fear. This is because of the anticipatory stress or worry that you are feeling. However, as you apply the procedures described later, you will become quite comfortable in that scene. Once you have mastered your fear there, you can proceed to another imagined scene which brings you a little closer to your fear. By moving along in a stepwise fashion, your unconscious mind gradually becomes accustomed to dealing with the lead up to *and* the actual feared situation itself. This process, known as imaginal or imagery desensitisation, is probably best carried out under the guidance of a therapist in the first instance. There are a few procedures though, that you can perform which will help you 'make contact' with the fear more easily.

Your automatic nervous system   It is useful for you to understand what happens inside your body when you become fearful. The first thing to realise is that you have two types of nervous system. One is involved in driving the voluntary organs such as your muscles and is known as the central nervous system. The other supplies the involuntary organs of your body: the lungs, heart, bowel, skin and glands. This second system is composed of two parts, the sympathetic and parasympathetic. The sympathetic system could be likened to an accelerator in a motorcar, whilst the parasympathetic is similar to a braking mechanism. Normal functioning of the involuntary organs depends upon a fine balance being maintained between these two branches. When confronted by a feared situation the sympathetic system overreacts (psychologists call this overarousal). A consequence of this overarousal of the sympathetic system is that certain organs become excessively stimulated. This may result in your experiencing unpleasant effects—a racing heart, rapid breathing, sweaty skin on the palms of your hands, dizziness and dryness of the mouth. It is the presence of these symptoms which often frightens people into believing that they are going to have a heart attack or fall unconscious.

Understanding the reason for your having any or all of these symptoms may be the first and most important step in setting out to treat your fear. Because of the wide variety of fears that are experienced by the population at large, it is not possible to describe all the procedures that can be applied in self-hypnotic treatment. I should like to reiterate that these are best learnt under the guidance of a therapist.

Using your relaxation cue   One way of desensitising yourself to your fear using self-hypnosis is to use a relaxation cue. With this technique, you first write in your work diary a hierarchy of scenes, i.e. a series of scenes connected with your fear starting from the least fearful, progressing in a step-wise fashion through increasingly more difficult ones until the final scene in which you are confronting the thing or situation that you fear. The fear or distress you experience in each scene can be gradually eased by the use of a relaxation cue mechanism. This acts as a 'prompt' for your unconscious mind, reminding you to relax even though you are being confronted by something that is stressful to you.

Having induced your self-hypnotic state, you can start your desensitising process by picturing yourself in the first scene in your hierarchy. This could be, for example, at home where you are surrounded by familiar things. Normally, you would feel very comfortable in that imagined scene but on this occasion, you are preparing to leave for . . .[insert here the feared situation]. Remember what it was like; think about it; imagine it and try to re-experience the scene as if you are actually there. As you do so, you may start to feel uncomfortable. You may notice your heart racing or your palms become sweaty. This discomfort shows that you are feeling anxious. If these feelings of anxiousness and nervousness appear, don't be unduly concerned for you can soon bring them under control.

You should continue to visualise yourself in the scene and, at the same time, concentrate on your breathing. As you breathe out each time think of the word 'calm'. Go on doing this with each exhalation until all your anxious feelings have settled. It may take many minutes before you achieve relief from your stress and it is important that you continue to use this procedure until you feel comfortable there.

Once your discomfort in that scene has settled, let that mental picture slip away from your mind and replace it with the next in your step-ladder of feared situations. Go through the whole process again and if you feel anxious, breathe away the tensions and think of the word 'calm' until you feel at ease. You will probably find that you have to do this over many sessions of self-hypnosis until, finally, you feel comfortable in the presence of the thing that you fear. Remember not to hurry this process— it takes quite a long time to desensitise yourself from your phobia.

The place of tranquillity Although many people find the relaxation cue an effective way of de-stressing themselves in an imagined fear situation, others prefer to 'lose' themselves into a tranquil scene whenever their fear levels rise. You may wonder about the wisdom of this. After all, you may ask, is it not true that in order to master *any* fear, you have to confront it rather than run away from it? This is certainly correct. But what you are planning to do in using this technique is to keep your stress to manageable levels whilst your unconscious mind learns to adjust to each fear exposure. The last thing you want to happen is for your fear to get out of control.

A technique that I have found suits many people is to picture yourself in the first of the step-ladder of scenes. You will probably notice that you are already feeling quite anxious and tense. You feel agitated at the thought of leaving for . . .[insert your feared situation] even though you are still at home surrounded by things familiar to you. So just for a while, change the scene in your mind. Picture yourself in a peaceful, tranquil scene: it may be one that you have experienced in the past or one that you simply imagine. Choose one where you can be completely at peace. If it was possible to be in a place where there was no anxiety, this would be the one. You may, for example, imagine going along your mental corridor into your own inner mental place.

Once you feel quite at ease again, and this may take quite a few minutes to achieve, you can return to your original scene. You will probably notice that you feel much more at ease than before, but if you still experience any anxiety or nervousness, just return to your own quiet haven until your stress has completely settled. You can go on repeating this procedure as often as you like until you feel very comfortable in your first scene. Having achieved control in that situation, you should move on to the next step in the fear hierarchy. Eventually you will be able to confront and feel at ease in the imagined fear situation itself.

What, in fact, you are doing in using these procedures is gradually introducing your mind to increasing degrees of fear. As it deals satisfactorily with each one, it feels more able to cope with a slightly harder scene until, finally, it is successful in staying with ease in the imagined fear situation.

Making contact with your fear Now that you can cope with your fear in the imaginal situation, you may wonder whether you can do so in real life. There is a wealth of anecdotal and research evidence[27] that shows that you can, but it must be emphasised that you should practise your new-found skills in real life. It is not sufficient to feel at ease as you imagine yourself coping with a formerly feared scene, whilst in the security of your own home. You *must* confront the same scene in everyday life for, after all, that is the purpose of these procedures.

At first you may find that doing this creates fresh anxieties. If this happens, just remember to use your relaxation cue. Think of 'calm' with each breath out until your stress has settled. This may take several minutes, but it is comforting to know that you can call upon this technique whenever and wherever you wish, instead of being overtaken by a feeling of blind panic.

Imagery rehearsal

There are many instances in life when we become tense and nervous, such as having to face up to a social situation or perform a task in front of others. This anticipatory stress serves to undermine our confidence and interfere with the efficiency of our performance. The thought of standing in front of a group of people and delivering a speech may prove daunting if not impossible to many. In a similar vein, many sportspeople feel that they are never as successful when performing in front of a crowd as they are when practicing.

Anxiety and fear arising from having to perform in public can be effectively dealt with using a technique of imagery rehearsal in self-hypnosis. The basic concept here is that of visualising yourself responding to the situation in an ideal, successful way. Try to imagine yourself and the anticipated scene in as much detail as you can. It may not be possible to do this if you have, for example, no prior experience of the venue. In this case, it may be necessary for you to draw on past experiences and 'see' yourself coping satisfactorily with these.

For this imagery technique to be successful, you will need to visualise yourself coping with a *variety* of possible difficulties that could arise. If you just imagined yourself, for example, standing up and successfully addressing a sales conference, you would not be making any allowance for the unexpected to happen. Audiovisual equipment does break down; microphones can fail to function, and not all audiences are friendly.

The art of imagery rehearsal in self-hypnosis lies in picturing yourself coping successfully with *all* contingencies that might arise. This may involve your being humorous, or learning to pause and assemble your facts when you are confronted by a tricky question from the audience. In spite of all your best laid plans, you may still encounter the unexpected. This will not prove to be any great problem, for your improved coping skills will easily help you to cope. It must be emphasised, however, that success depends on daily reinforcement of these imagery techniques for at least a week before the event.

CHAPTER FIVE

COPING WITH WORK-RELATED STRESS

It is a fact of life that the majority of us are constantly confronted by a wide variety of pressures associated with the maintenance of an acceptable standard of living. Raising and educating a family or paying off a mortgage on your home can be significantly stressful in themselves, but over and above this, many people have burdens to carry at work that create such high levels of stress that their physical and mental health is undermined.

What are the factors in your job situation which might damage your health? They can be many and varied and it is obviously necessary for you to be able to identify those that especially apply to you before you can learn to cope with them.

Job satisfaction

If you could divide up your day so that you could achieve ideal health, you would probably split it roughly into thirds: one for work, one for sleep, and one for leisure and other activities. Now clearly this is a counsel of perfection and, in the normal course of events, a situation that few can achieve. Generally, it is the work segment which creates the most demands and this has the effect of unbalancing other aspects of life.

Being unhappy in your work will invariably cause you to become stressed. Lack of job satisfaction can stem from several factors. Obviously if you are in a position which proves too demanding, or is beyond your capabilities, stress will soon enter the picture. On the other hand, having too little to do, or working in an area which is not challenging enough for you, can prove equally stressful.[28] Every job involves a certain amount of repetition, but usually there will be periods of stimulation. Problems tend to arise when there is a lack of variation, sheer monotony being the source of stress. As one of my patients so graphically described it, 'When I wake up each morning to the realisation that I am faced by another round of household chores, I feel I want to scream'.

If job dissatisfaction is so much a cause of stress, why is it that more people do not make the necessary change in their work scene, or modify their lifestyle to offset the tedium? The answer to this question lies in that vital personality factor called self-esteem. Feeling locked into a job that you are not enjoying not only creates stress but also undermines self-worth. As self-esteem diminishes there tends to be a corresponding increase in a person's fear of failure, fear that if they make a change they may again be faced by the same lack of success that they are currently experiencing. This prospect can be daunting, to say the least. In a sense, it becomes a case of 'the devil you know is better than the one you don't know.'

What such a person will be failing to realise is that all of us possess a particular personality makeup which makes us more suitable for one line of work than another. One person, for example, may have personality traits which are best suited to a managerial role involving the control of a large group of workers. Another may possess quite different qualities and prefer to work alone or in a small group environment. Metaphorically, being a square peg in a round hole can be stressful.

Working against the clock

Time constraints, too, can be very stress inducing and if they are a major feature can lead to loss of job satisfaction. Fortunately for most of us, having to complete certain projects in a limited time only occurs in a sporadic fashion, but even short bursts of increased demands on time can have damaging effects on health. This was demonstrated in a study carried out on accountants, which showed their blood cholesterol levels rose and they had an increased tendency to blood clotting when they were under pressure to complete tax returns at the end of the financial year. Another study showed that raised blood pressure was more prevalent in air traffic controllers who worked with high density traffic.[29] All of these health factors can significantly increase your chances of having a heart attack.

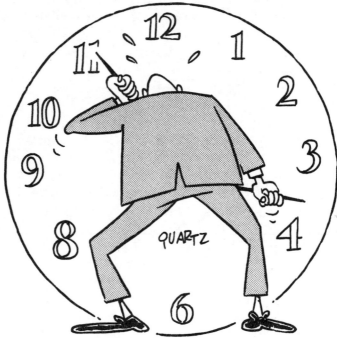

Time constraints can be stress inducing

Ideally, you should aim to pace yourself so as to reduce workload peaks and troughs. To do so you will need to have an adequate and committed staff, each member of which is set well-defined goals and priorities. In such an environment it is possible to achieve high performance with a minimal amount of stress, irrespective of how much work there is to be done.

The demands of responsibility

The principal goal for most of us in our work sphere is to be successful, but how we view success is a very personal matter. Some see it as having a large income, or achieving a position of some standing in an organisation. For others, success stems from the enjoyment and sense of achievement which they derive from work. Whatever criteria you use, success generally goes hand-in-hand with promotion and this, unfortunately, can sometimes create a whole new set of problems.

While the increased responsibility that promotion brings may prove to be very stimulating and challenging, and can bring out the best in you, some find responsibility onerous and thus extremely stressful.

One of the major features of this stress is an increased tendency to worry about things associated with work. A patient, recently promoted to area manager of a computer software company, described to me how he woke up in the early hours each morning, his mind overwhelmed by concerns about things which had to be done and problems that had to be confronted. Even though logic told him that there was little he could do at that moment to deal with such matters, he found it impossible to halt the flow of negative thoughts. What he had developed was the condition of anticipatory stress, otherwise known as worry. This anticipatory anxiety served to fuel his overall stress picture, and he admitted that his work efficiency was suffering as a result.

The fear of failure

The drop in performance levels that results from stress may induce other concerns, especially fears of job loss. In the competitive world in which we live organisations demand maximum efficiency from their staff, and therefore failure to perform satisfactorily is likely to place your job in jeopardy. You might think that such a sword of Damocles hanging over you would act as a stimulus to improve your performance, but because stress becomes intensified it generally has the opposite effect.

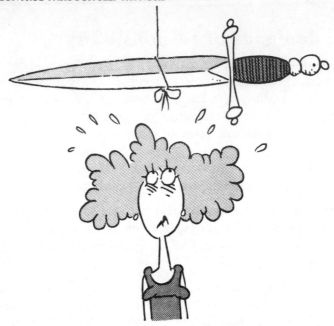

Fear of failure can hang over us like the sword of Damocles

The importance of self-esteem

A feature of any work organisation is the need for constant staff appraisal. Depending on your performance ratings, you can be promoted, demoted or lose your job. Most of us accept that constant assessment by others in more senior positions is a necessary prerequisite if we are to gain promotion, and if the organisation for which we work is to function efficiently. There are those, however, who find this accountability to be a major source of stress, especially if self-esteem is already at a low ebb.

Good self-esteem is a most valuable attribute. Although it was discussed in detail in Chapter 1, it is of such importance, especially in determining how successful you are in your work, that it is worth reiterating its major features. If you have good self-esteem (also known as self-worth or self-efficacy) you will be able to enter into any aspect of your life with a realistic expectation of success. You will have a sound belief in yourself and in your own abilities. Along with this, you will feel a constant need to develop these still further. If, at times, you are unable to achieve the things you set out to do, you will be able to come to terms with this quite easily, without necessarily feeling that you have failed.

If you have a feeling of self-worth, you will be able to accept criticism in a constructive fashion rather than 'taking it to heart'. By the same token, you will feel comfortable expressing your own views and opinions whenever you consider them to be justified, instead of 'holding back' in case you upset someone. In short, you will have a sense of mental independence which enables you to deal with people and situations in a positive manner. Not surprisingly, these features will be recognised by those around you, especially work colleagues, and will influence their reactions to you.

Contrast this with a loss of these qualities, one of the features associated with stress. You become unsure in your judgements, entertaining all manner of self-doubts, and this results in your being unable to be as directive and as competent as you would wish. Others around you may interpret this as a sign that you are ill-equipped for the demands of your job and so your chances of advancement will be affected.

The answer to low self-esteem lies in reducing your stress levels. You will then be able to perceive things quite differently, instead of approaching job situations in a negative frame of mind. Through the use of appropriate suggestions and imagery in self-hypnosis, your self-esteem will progressively improve to the extent that you will start to realise your own potential. You will begin to recognise areas of success unfolding in your life, and once this process has been initiated it tends to become self-propagating.

Do you have a social phobia?

Another facet of increased responsibility that you may find stressful is having to address groups of people, such as board members, trainee staff or members of other organisations. Some people find these experiences enjoyable and stimulating, but others dread the possibility of having to stand up and address groups of people, be they small or large. This qualifies as a social phobia or fear, and can be a major source of stress, even for someone who is quite competent in every other aspect of their business life.

Such a fear can arise for several reasons. First, it can be associated with low self-esteem. Where this is the case, you become overly concerned with what other people may be thinking of you and of the things you have to say. You wonder whether they will be critical of you and whether you are really the right person to be addressing them.

Negative thinking or self-talk concerned with worry about making a mistake can be another major cause of this phobia. This is best summarised by a patient's description of his thoughts before giving an address: 'I know my field quite well, but what if I "choke" when I stand up? Wouldn't it be embarrassing if I can't get my words out, or lose my place? The group would think I am a real idiot.' Such negative thought patterns can only lead to your becoming tense and stressed, and will set in train the very effects you fear.

A third possible reason for this fear is concern over being stared at, or more precisely of eye contact. Obviously, an audience is going to look at you if you are speaking to them, and yet it is this aspect which some find the most unsettling.

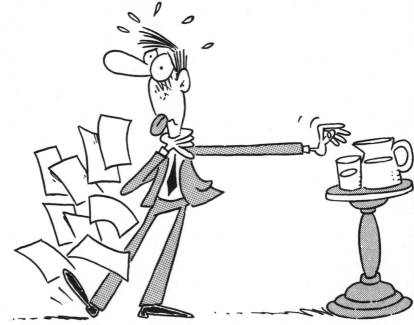

Fears such as addressing a group can be overcome through
self-hypnosis

Michael was a perfect example of someone who suffered from a social phobia. He was a thirty-five-year-old executive who had been appointed national sales manager for a major computer company. His promotion through the sales field had been rapid, for he was zealous and hardworking. He had a sound educational background and had no difficulty in addressing colleagues when at a lower level of sales management.

One of his first roles as a senior executive was to address a large meeting of sales staff, many of whom were from overseas. Prior to that major sales conference, he started to dwell on all sorts of negative thoughts, and entertained doubts as to whether he was capable of addressing the group. He worried about how he would sound when he spoke, and hoped his mind 'wouldn't go blank'. As the conference drew closer, the greater his fears became.

When he stood up to address the meeting he felt tremulous and nervous. He was unsure of what to do with his hands and was concerned that the audience would notice they were shaking. His mouth felt dry, his voice wavered and his thought patterns became erratic. In spite of having put a great deal of preparation into the talk, Michael knew that his delivery and demeanour fell far short of what he would have wished.

This traumatic experience had a devastating effect on his self-esteem and from that point on even addressing small groups of salespeople became a major task, one which he avoided whenever possible. Unbeknown to him, this avoidance strategy only served to intensify his fear.

Initially he sought hypnotic treatment for his fear problem, but in time he became adept at using self-hypnotic suggestions and imagery in order to prepare himself for each talk he had to make. In his work diary he wrote a list of all the possible difficulties that could arise and then, in self-hypnosis, imagined himself coping with each in turn. Before bringing a self-hypnotic session to a close, he made a point of spending several minutes visualising himself talking about his topic in an easy, relaxed attitude. Practising these techniques regularly over a period of six months finally enabled him to speak to any group quite free from fear and tension.

You and your work colleagues

In a work environment, anyone in a managerial position, whether as a top-level executive or in middle management, will need a two-pronged approach to stress. First, it will be necessary for you to reduce the stress in yourself which stems from carrying out a challenging job and, second, you will need to help employees reduce the stress they may be experiencing at work. To be a successful manager you will need to be in constant touch with personnel under your control, and be willing to reorganise work loads when these are seen to be excessive.

It is little wonder, given these requirements, that supervisors and middle managers, in particular, become excessively stressed. They often feel pulled in one direction by the demands imposed by managers above them, and in another by the problems and demands of employees under their control. This conflict of allegiance is not restricted to the business world: it has also been shown to lead to stress in the teaching profession and the police force.

In a management situation, the effect of stress on an individual is not always readily apparent. Sometimes it can be recognised by changes in behaviour. Thus, it may manifest itself by a staff member making aggressive, inappropriate statements, or having angry outbursts at meetings. Others may show irritability or discourtesy and frequently, stress leads to a lack of harmony in the executive team.

Clearly there are many aspects of your working life that cause you to become stressed, and generally they are associated with factors you cannot change, short of choosing a different occupation or way of life. What *is* important is how you deal with these work issues and stressors. If they remain unchecked, they are likely to have a damaging effect on both your psychological and physical health.

STRESS AND YOUR HEART

Although stress can affect virtually any of your body's organs, the ones that are usually of most concern are the heart and blood vessels. The prospect of being incapacitated or, worse still, dying of a heart attack or stroke, is understandably frightening to most people. All too often the stress that leads to these disorders is work related. It makes good sense, therefore, to consider the various ways in which stress can link up with other factors to affect your circulatory system.

The 'other factors' that put you at greater risk of developing coronary heart disease or having a heart attack are your personality make up, a family history of heart problems, raised blood pressure, increased blood lipids (fats), obesity and smoking. If stress is superimposed on any of these, it can greatly reduce your chances of maintaining good health. Once you have an understanding of these, you should be better able to take the necessary steps to protect yourself from heart disease.

Your personality make up

One of the interesting facets of the human race is that no two people are identical in physical make up. Even so-called identical twins have slight differences that distinguish one from the other. In the same way, it is fascinating to consider that no two people have identical personalities. This genetic curiosity ensures that, in any given situation, each of us is likely to respond differently.

Medical researchers and psychologists have studied the relationship between individuals' personalities and their predisposition to certain disorders, in particular, heart disease. Out of these studies came the terms type A and type B personalities.[30]

Type A personalities are depicted as being driving, aggressive people who are easily aroused to hostility and are stimulated by challenging situations and events. They have difficulty sitting still and 'doing nothing', and invariably are involved in several projects at the same time. For this reason they are highly productive, are rarely sick, and almost never have cause to visit their doctor. Even their leisure activities such as jogging, squash or tennis are pursued with the same degree of intensity and competitiveness that they bring to their office.

Type B personalities, on the other hand, are more inclined to listen and deliberate before acting. They are phlegmatic, philosophical and less impulsive than their type A counterparts. Leisure activities and hobbies usually form an important part

of their lifestyle but are conducted in a less competitive way—
one that enables them to detach themselves more easily from
the stressful situations of life.

Personality and heart disease

You should be interested in your personality type because of
the relationship that exists between it and the possibility of
having a heart attack. Coronary heart disease is not only
frightening, but it can greatly interfere with your ability to
work, or even perform everyday activities. In Australia in 1977,
315 men per 100 000 and 241 women per 100 000 population
died as the result of heart disease, which indicates the scale
of the problem.

Apart from the severely disruptive effects that coronary heart
disease has on an individual, it is worth considering the effect
that temporary or permanent loss of an executive has on an
organisation. Business expertise and contacts are acquired over
many years and the loss of these skills can be financially
incalculable for a company.

Research has shown that type A personalities are much more
likely than type B to suffer a heart attack, especially at a younger
age.[31] The critical behavioural factor that seems to be at the
centre of the type A's predisposition to heart disease is their
tendency towards hostility and unexpressed anger. But not all
the news is bad for type A individuals, for it has been shown
that their recovery rate after a heart attack is as good as that
of type Bs.[32] Obviously, not everyone falls neatly under the
mantle of being either type A or type B, people usually being
a mixture of both. Nevertheless, if you have a preponderance
of type A features, you are likely to be more prone to heart
disease.

Is heart disease in your family?

It has been shown, quite clearly, that many of the health
problems you may be experiencing occur because you have
inherited a predisposition to the disease. Coronary heart disease
is a classic example of this. If, say, your father or uncle had
a heart attack at a relatively early age, this puts you at a much
greater risk of suffering the same fate.

Even if you have an inherited predisposition to coronary heart disease, however, this does not imply that you should turn yourself into an invalid or wait for the inevitable to occur. Whether you have heart trouble or not may well depend upon what steps you take to change certain patterns of behaviour in your life—in other words, the moves you make to minimise all other factors that put you at risk of having a heart attack. Changes in behaviour centre on the need to reduce stress; others require you to modify other aspects of your life. All these factors are, of course, interrelated but it is interesting to note that, irrespective of which factor you consider, stress always seems to be lurking in the background.

The bad effects of raised blood pressure

In normal health, your blood pressure varies depending on whether you are sitting or standing, exercising or at rest, stressed or relaxed, and also on your age. Usually your physician will record blood pressure readings when you are at rest, for these give the most accurate indications of normality.

But why is it so important to know whether your blood pressure is raised? The principal reason is that high blood pressure, or hypertension, is considered to be both one of the most important accelerating factors and, perhaps, *the* most correctable aspect in the development of coronary heart disease.[33]

While the genes you inherit may bring about high blood pressure, stressful work situations have also been shown to be a major cause of such problems.[34] If stress and emotion are such potent factors in raising your blood pressure, it would be reasonable to assume that the use of self-hypnosis should reverse the process, and indeed it does.[35]

Stress and blood clotting

Sustained stress can also interfere with the normal blood clotting mechanisms. It causes the blood to clot quicker and this, in turn, leads to a relative thickening of the blood as it flows around the body.[36] If the coronary or heart arteries are already narrowed because of a thickening of their walls (a condition called arteriosclerosis) the thickened blood is likely to block the vessel, affecting the supply of blood to the heart. In the absence of a good blood supply, the heart muscle can no longer function as it should and it is this that causes a heart attack.

HOW TO PREVENT HEART DISEASE

Even though stress is one of the major villains of the piece, it is not the only factor to be acknowledged if you are to stay healthy. Other patterns of lifestyle and behaviour can also play significant roles.

The importance of exercise

Regular exercise and a satisfactory diet are two factors which cannot be ignored. Over the past decade or so there has been a veritable explosion in the taking of exercise of all kinds— jogging, aerobics, dancing and cycling being but a few examples. This can probably be attributed to a combination of factors. Health and medical authorities are, at last, starting to promote the concept of preventative medicine, the aim being to stop diseases occurring. People throughout the world, too, are becoming more aware of the need to involve themselves in their *own* health programs. In earlier days people were surprisingly unprepared to take responsibility for looking after their health.

It is often the teachings of a 'guru' that galvanises people into action. Take jogging, for example. One of the earliest proponents of this form of exercise was Dr Kenneth Cooper. He suggested that jogging was something that was suitable for everyone, provided they went through a graduated build-up. His main proposition was that jogging helps to protect the heart from coronary disease and also promotes a sense of well-being. These views were based on sound research data, and anybody interested in developing an exercise program could do no better than consult Cooper's *The New Aerobics*.[37]

For every person who becomes dedicated to the exercise cause, however, it is probably true to say that an equal number view the prospect with reluctance or even downright distaste. Not surprisingly, they question whether the benefits of exercise justify the amount of effort and time invested. This issue has also preoccupied doctors and physiologists for some time, and although there are those who hold reservations about the benefits of exercise, the majority support the notion that it is of immense value to you.

Psychological benefits of fitness

You may think of exercise as a means of protecting you from heart disease, but you should not underestimate its other benefits. There could be no better way of expressing this than 'Nearly all individuals find that an increase in habitual physical activity will produce an increase in physical (and perhaps mental) vigour, stamina and enthusiasm and that it may enhance creativity and optimism as well'.[38]

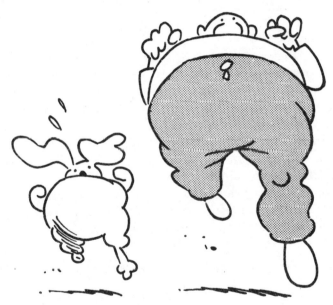

Jogging or other exercise helps keep us relaxed as well as physically healthy

Many of us find that regular exercise acts as a form of tranquilliser, releasing the tensions and stresses of the day. At first it was thought that this was because exercise afforded us 'time out' during which we could detach ourselves from the cares and concerns of the day. This may indeed be partly true, but a more scientific explanation is that exercise causes our body to release into the bloodstream large amounts of tranquilliser-like substances called endorphins.[1] This could account for the 'improvement in personal self-image, *joie-de-vivre*, and tolerance to stress that is reported by many, but not all, who invest their energies in an endurance-enhancing activity program'.[38] It is clear, therefore, that even solely as a means of stress management and coping better with life, the taking of exercise is fully justified.

Fitness and your body

While regular exercise helps reduce blood pressure and thus reduces strain on the heart, it should be emphasised that if you have high blood pressure there are certain precautionary measures you *must* take before launching yourself on the fitness trail.

The first of these is to have a thorough medical check-up from your doctor, which may entail your undergoing a stress test. A stress test is not related to stress as applied throughout this book but involves your walking or jogging on a treadmill, or cycling on a bicycle ergometer whilst tracings of your heart's activity are being recorded. This enables your physician to determine whether you can start an exercise program with complete safety. Even in the absence of raised blood pressure, it would be unwise for any person over the age of thirty-five years, who has not been engaged in regular exercise, to embark on getting fit without first being tested in this way. An ounce of prevention is far better than a pound of cure.

How exercise affects your blood fats

Another way in which exercise can benefit your body is by changing the levels of your blood fats or lipids. Usually these are measured in the laboratory in terms of levels of cholesterol and triglycerides, which are carried in the bloodstream as lipoproteins. As part of your medical check-up your doctor is therefore likely to take a blood sample for blood fat levels to be measured.

There are two types of lipoproteins: high density (HDL) and low density lipoproteins (LDL). The high density ones have the effect of protecting your blood vessels (these are the 'good guys') whilst the low density cause a silting-up effect or atheroma to develop (these are the 'bad guys'). In unfit males the LDL fraction is usually higher than the HDL and consequently there is a greater danger of blockage in the heart or brain arteries. Regular exercise can cause the HDL levels to rise, thus protecting your blood vessels and heart.

I specifically point to males being affected in this way. Nature has been a great deal kinder to females for, normally, their HDL levels are in excess of the LDL, and this may be one reason why women are less prone to heart attacks.

Why you should quit smoking   One of the many harmful effects smoking has is to increase the LDL and decrease the HDL in both men and women. So, if you are a woman who smokes, you are breaking down one of nature's protective barriers.[39]

Smokers have a four-fold greater incidence of heart attacks than non-smokers,[40] and 'cigarette smokers have a significantly higher incidence of stroke than non-smokers, regardless of the number of cigarettes smoked'.[41] If you add to these the increased danger of developing lung cancer, emphysema, and cancer of the larynx and oesophagus, there would seem to be little to recommend this poisonous habit. Health authorities throughout the world have tried to bring this to the attention of the public but it still remains a significant health problem. Obviously, there are a great many reasons why people smoke, but one that cannot be ignored is the effect of stress, for people smoke more when they are under pressure. The improvement in your self-image that stems from both the reduction of stress through self-hypnosis and regular exercise, can be a major help in overcoming 'tobaccomania'.[42]

So you are overweight

One of the major health problems confronting people in the more affluent countries of the world is obesity, and yet few of us enjoy being flabby. Why then do we put on excessive weight? Obviously either we eat too much or we eat the wrong types of food.

Once past the age of twenty-five years, your need for a high kilojoule intake diminishes, for no longer are you using up energy in growing and laying down new tissues in your body. Because of this, your food requirements should be determined by how much energy you have to expend each day in your work and other activities. If you are in a sedentary job, such as working in an office, you will need to eat far less than if you are performing heavy manual labour. Unfortunately, whatever our actual kilojoule requirements, we tend to eat more, rather than less, the more successful we are.

Apart from the amount of food you eat, the types of food you eat also clearly have a significant bearing on weight. This is the age of fast food and take-aways, and these must come high on your list of 'forbidden foods' if you are to keep control of your weight. If you are overweight the chances are that you are eating more fatty foods (including oils) than you realise. Fast foods are inclined to be heavily laden with these substances.

Why you overeat

Why people overeat is a complex issue. The psychological factor most commonly associated with overweight and a poor eating pattern is low self-esteem, but whether this occurs as the result of being obese, or as a factor in causing a person to eat too much is not always easy to define. It is certainly a truism that most people who suffer these problems usually have a poor body image.[43] Stress, too, plays its part. People tend to eat more when stressed or unhappy, as if food acts as a solace to them. Unfortunately, having raided the larder, feelings of guilt invariably ensue and add to the whole stressful cycle.

The business lunch

If you are in an executive position, you may well be confronted with an additional burden in trying to control your weight— the business lunch. While it may be a very necessary aspect of life, being a forum for discussing matters with colleagues, it can prove to be something of a *bête-noir* weight-wise unless you are consciously taking care over what you eat.

Your weight difficulties can be further compounded if your lunch is accompanied by a liberal supply of alcohol. Apart from the excessive kilojoule content of alcohol, it can add to your health woes by significantly raising your blood pressure.[44] On both counts, there would seem to be ample justification for keeping a weather-eye on your alcohol intake.

A guide to weight control

Keeping control over your weight is often no more than a matter of commonsense, given that it involves not eating too much and eating the right types of food. This may sound simplistic, but because your eating behaviour is often influenced by stress and social habits, such a regime may be difficult at first to implement.

Your first line of attack should be directed towards eating the correct foods. Two large studies, one carried out by the American College of Physicians and the other by the Royal College of Physicians in Britain, have resulted in the provision of certain guidelines.

—Fats are to be avoided as much as possible. Eating fatty foods causes you to become fat.
—Weight loss is a slow process. It is quite easy for you to gain weight but much harder to lose it. You should aim to lose weight gradually, over a long period of time. Bear in mind that crash diets are temporary phenomena and no one can live indefinitely on one.
—There is a need for you to establish a correct pattern of eating. The foods that have been shown to be of greatest benefit in losing weight and, more importantly, staying at the desired weight, are the complex carbohydrates: vegetables, fruit, pasta and wholegrain dishes. This type of fare does not need to be boring and there are countless cookbooks available which will provide you with a variety of interesting recipes that will stimulate your taste buds.

Your weight control graph

Modification of any behaviours, including those associated with eating, requires you to constantly monitor your progress. This helps to reinforce the newly established patterns of eating and also ensures that they are effective.

The use of a weight graph will enable you to assess your progress and thus adjust your eating patterns in order to maintain a gradual weight loss. As an example of this, assume that your present weight is 100 kg. You may consider your ideal and realistic weight should be 75 kg. Draw up a graph as depicted below:

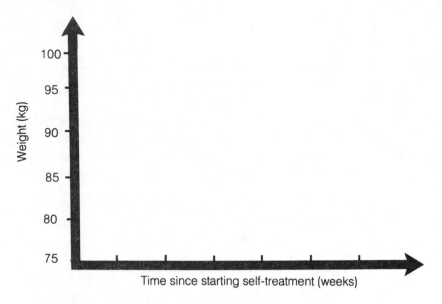

Time since starting self-treatment (weeks)

Record your weight on the same day each week and weigh yourself unclothed first thing in the morning (to eliminate variable factors such as fluid retention). Monitoring your progress in this way will motivate you to reach your goal. If there is a plateau effect or temporary rise in weight at any stage, you should not be discouraged. It indicates you are wandering from your eating plan and this should stimulate you to correct this situation as soon as possible.

Stress and your eating pattern

Self-hypnosis can help you to reduce stress and provide you with a means of 'reprogramming' your mind to enjoy your new eating habits. Negative self-talk (see Chapter 4) will undermine your good intentions to lose weight: self-statements such as 'I'm not very strong-willed: I find it so hard to resist eating cakes' *must* be replaced by positive coping suggestions if you are to succeed. It is far better for you to think 'I know I have had difficulties with my eating in the past and do enjoy cakes [here you are recognising the reality of the situation] but I know these are going to add to my weight problem. Instead, I will enjoy eating an apple (or go and involve myself in some other activity) and will look forward to this in the future'. These coping suggestions can be constantly reinforced in self-hypnosis and, over a period of time, you will notice that they lead to progressive changes in your eating behaviours.

The importance of sleep

A problem that commonly arises when you are stressed is difficulty in going to sleep, or remaining asleep all night. This may arise because you are unable to detach yourself from business or professional worries—it is as if you cannot 'switch off your mind'. It is little wonder that sleep becomes difficult under these circumstances. Sometimes, too, sleep problems arise because business commitments entail travelling away from home and having to spend nights in a series of strange situations.

Whatever the cause, inadequate sleep can seriously impair the way you function in life by not allowing you to 'recharge your mental batteries'. In such situations you wake up feeling lethargic and far from ready to face the work demands of the day. Under such circumstances a vicious cycle can be set up in which you worry about *not* sleeping. Inevitably this anticipatory concern only serves to intensify the problem.

How to approach sleep

Because sound, restful sleep is so important if you are to perform to capacity, you need to develop techniques which will help you relax when you go to bed. The first step you must take, if you are to break down the fear of not sleeping, is to look upon bed as a place where you can relax. Think of how pleasant it is to snuggle down between the bedsheets; of how quiet and peaceful it is. You may find it beneficial to take a milk drink before retiring for it has been shown that tryptophan, one of the constituents of milk, helps promote sleep.[45] Avoid tea or coffee because of their stimulant qualities. Some people resort to alcohol in the mistaken belief that it will sedate them. Although it can have an immediate soporific action, you may find that you waken in the early hours and have great difficulty returning to sleep.

Self-hypnosis as a prelude to sleep

Although you should generally avoid using self-hypnosis in bed, the one exception to this rule is where you wish to use it as a lead-in to sleep. Going through your favoured induction procedures may, in itself, be sufficient to induce drowsiness. However, if you are still awake at the end of these, you need not be concerned for you still have a number of ways of taking yourself off into the arms of Morpheus.

Without terminating self-hypnosis, suggest to yourself that you are going to turn into the position in which you normally sleep, and that in a little while your relaxation is going to flow gently into a deep, peaceful sleep. If intrusive thoughts about the office or work still bother you, let your mind drift off into pleasant imagery. Some like to imagine themselves involved in active imagery—playing a game of tennis or golf, or walking along a beach. Others prefer to visualise themselves resting somewhere quiet, such as a lovely garden.

Another valuable aid to sleep is to take yourself into your inner mental place. Picture yourself walking along a beautiful corridor in your mind until you come to a door that leads to your own inner mental place. As you open the door and step inside, you find yourself in a most beautiful, tranquil place— one where nothing can intrude on your peace of mind. As you close the door behind you, feel as though you are shutting out all the problems and concerns of work and life, so that you can enjoy exploring that special place in your mind in a leisurely fashion. Rarely does this technique fail to help achieve sleep, even in those who have been plagued by insomnia.

Are you a workaholic?

Illness in a loved one, financial troubles, moving house, death of a close family member and sexual difficulties are but a few of the many major life stressors that can affect us.[46] In the case of business executives and professional people, stress often arises because of the constancy and intensity of work demands. Such people become so embroiled in work that it dominates their whole life, becoming an addiction. Workaholic is the term generally used for this sort of person.

If you would like to know whether you are a workaholic, answer yes or no to the following statements, according to what most accurately describes your typical actions or feelings. The results may surprise you. I am indebted to Kitty Vivekananda for her permission to use and adapt the questionnaire, which was taken from the article 'Helping yourself cope with stress', published in *Medical Observer*.

1. I feel guilty if I take time for myself to relax or do nothing. yes/no
2. I find it difficult to separate work from my personal life. yes/no
3. I can't switch off from work problems when I go home. yes/no
4. I feel at a loss when the activity of the day comes to an end. yes/no
5. I don't have time to see family or close friends. yes/no
6. At dinner parties I have little else to talk about but my work. yes/no
7. I pride myself on being hard-driving and ambitious. yes/no

Yes responses to these questions indicate the extent to which you are a workaholic personality type. While a certain amount of stress is productive, useful and even exciting, in the long run excessive stress becomes counterproductive.

While we are young, we take for granted our energy and health. At mid-life, if work has been an all-consuming obsession, workaholics often suffer from burnout and disillusionment about their achievements. They find themselves asking questions like 'Is this all there is?'

Such people draw their self-esteem primarily from work, neglecting other areas of their lives such as relaxation, non-competitive activities, hobbies, relationships and doing nothing.

One technique you may find helpful is that suggested by a business acquaintance. He draws a line through each Sunday in his diary and writes 'playday' across the page. By doing this, he is giving himself permission to take the day off from all business matters and ensuring that he has no need to feel guilty when he involves himself in other activities.

Taking time out from business or professional pressures is an art that can be cultivated. Some years ago there was a delightful programme screened on television concerning the barges on the canals of Europe. A gentle old man lived near the canal bank and spent the greater part of each day gazing at the barges as they slowly made their way past. His inner tranquillity was obvious when he said 'Now is the time, time to learn the gentle art of doing nothing'. Perhaps your object should be to learn this gentle art.

As mentioned earlier, another way to release stress is through the use of regular exercise such as jogging. But if you find taking exercise too demanding or unacceptable to you, do not despair. Even digging the garden, mowing the lawn or painting a room can be useful ways of releasing 'emotional steam'. They all have the effect of distracting your attention from the work scene for a while.

The questionnaire continues:

8. I wake up each morning feeling I have not slept properly. yes/no
9. I feel generally run down and tired most of the time. yes/no
10. I find it difficult to relax. yes/no
11. I am becoming more forgetful about appointments, deadlines and personal possessions. yes/no
12. I am working harder and harder but accomplishing less. yes/no
13. I frequently get short-tempered over little things. yes/no
14. I am smoking/drinking/eating more than I used to. yes/no

Watch out if you answered yes to these statements, for they are indicators of overload, stress or burnout. This is an important time to decide who and what is important in your life. Take up some sports, hobbies, exercises, or personal development courses. There are many excellent courses conducted by evening colleges, workers' education associations and university unions.

Learn to relax using your self-hypnosis. Set aside fifteen to twenty minutes each day as *your* special time to relax your mind and body. See it as being an important way for you to 'recharge your mental batteries'. Those moments of peace will help you gain a much better perspective on life and on your work.

Give yourself some quiet time on your own each day to think and unwind: every minute does not have to be productive. Read novels, or go to films and exhibitions to broaden your areas of interest and topics of conversation. Spend time having fun and developing relationships with your spouse, children and friends. Do not be discouraged if they fail to respond immediately to *your* changes. Just remember it takes time to develop relationships.

15. I frequently get irritated or impatient with other people and events. yes/no
16. I pride myself on getting things done faster than other people. yes/no
17. I frequently feel critical and angry with others for their inability to hold up their end. yes/no

An affirmative answer to these statements reveals that you may set high standards for other people, but of course they may not always live up to your high expectations. If you do not modify or compromise your expectations, you are doomed to stress-related disappointment and resentment.

Communicate your expectations clearly to others, rather than expecting them to read your mind. In a situation of frustration, assess whether you have any control over it. If you cannot do anything about it, getting worried or irritated is simply a waste of energy. Try to develop a sense of humour and be prepared to shrug off minor irritations.

18. In order to be acceptable as a person, I have to be the best in all things. yes/no

19. No matter what success I achieve, I still do not feel good about myself. yes/no
20. I feel despondent even when small things go wrong. yes/no
21. I worry about what others think of me. yes/no
22. Life has lost its enjoyment and fun. yes/no
23. I feel as though I don't want to hear about other people's problems. yes/no

If you agreed with these statements it indicates an over-emphasis on achievement and success as the major source of self-esteem and worth.

All of us need to be loved and valued unconditionally, not just when we are being useful, helpful and successful. A fear of discovering your inadequacy, weakness, vulnerability and loneliness can keep you chained to a treadmill of achievement, even when it is no longer satisfying. Acknowledging your humanity can be a great source of creativity, compassion, sensitivity and love. Allow yourself to 'just be' instead of continually trying to be busy. Develop relationships where you are *not* the expert or helper. Remind yourself that you do not always have to be right in everything you do.

24. I maintain appearances that I am an independent person. yes/no
25. I turn away support and assistance even when I have need. yes/no
26. I expect others to guess or know what I want, without my asking. yes/no

You may be the sort of person who finds it hard to discuss problems and concerns, and especially when you are stressed. Remember that when you 'bottle up' your worries you add to your feelings of frustration and stress. Be prepared to talk over your concerns with someone you trust—your spouse, a close friend, a parent or your doctor. Talking things over will often help you to stand back from the problem and bring it into perspective. At best, it will help you resolve it. At the very least, it will stop you distorting or magnifying it in your mind.

27. I support and help others even when I don't wish to. yes/no
28. I don't assert myself in negotiations. yes/no
29. I place unrealistic expectations on myself that result in overextension. yes/no
30. I try to anticipate other people's needs ahead of time. yes/no
31. I have trouble delegating tasks to other people. yes/no

If you answered yes to any of these statements, you have trouble being assertive. Assertiveness includes the ability to say no to requests for your time or effort, and being able to ask for help. An inability to put limits on your time, energy and responsibility causes considerable stress.

People who cannot say no to demand, usually want to avoid offence, conflict or unpopularity. Unassertive people feel they have lost control of their lives, feel burdened, resentful, imposed upon or live with the illusion they are indispensable.

Evaluate whether you *have* to meet a given demand or request. If you choose to turn down a request don't say it in an angry, sarcastic or aggressive way. Use a relaxed voice and give brief reasons for declining the request. For example: 'I would really like to do that but I won't be able to because I am already working two nights this week'.

When delegating tasks to others communicate your expectations or request clearly. Again, watch *how* you ask. 'Why do I always have to do everything?' is not very clear communication. Be specific about what you want and when you want it done. If the other person is unable to meet these conditions, be prepared to negotiate and compromise.

After the job has been done, check it and thank the delegatee for doing the work. If it is appropriate, comment on how well the job was done, or make suggestions on how the job could be done more easily, better or faster the next time. If there is no one to whom to delegate, consider employing someone to do it.

32. I always respond to things when they occur. yes/no
33. Time is out of my control. yes/no

People are often more conscious of budgeting money than time, which is also a limited and precious resource. Time management is an important strategy in reducing stress and increasing efficiency.

Write down goals that have to be achieved: (a) immediately; (b) in the short-term future; (c) in the long-term future; or (d) are nice possibilities if you have the time and the resources.

Each day, set aside ten minutes to establish priorities and write them down. Don't feel pressured to handle everything immediately. Set aside time later when you will deal with problems. Also, try to avoid over-committing yourself.

Set aside uninterrupted time for tasks that require your attention. If you have trouble completing tasks, set deadlines in your diary.

There is little doubt that the constant pressures of work can prove damaging to your wellbeing and quality of life. Quite often, these work stresses are intertwined with poor lifestyle behaviours and only serve to add to your health problems. Correcting these, as I hope I have indicated, is none too difficult once you realise what the problems are and how they can be combatted.

The need to take care of yourself cannot be overemphasised, for as Carruthers and Taggart[47] so aptly expressed it: 'Reducing the incidence of coronary heart disease is available without the need for any new scientific miracles. If the population could be induced to eat and smoke less, *reduce their stress levels*, and take more of the right sort of exercise, one could confidently expect to decrease the number of heart attacks to a fraction of their present level' (my emphasis).

STRESS IN SPORT

Competition between individuals has always been seen as an important factor in their development. This behaviour is not restricted to humans, for it can also be observed in other members of the animal kingdom. You have only to watch young lions or monkeys playing and competing with each other to see how valuable this is as part of the animals' learning processes. From their play, they learn certain skills which may ensure their future survival.

From primitive beginnings a wide variety of sports has developed—competitive situations in which individuals can pit their skills against others. The desire to do well and win has led, as one would expect, to the progressive refinement of techniques and the development of special skills. New techniques of training, improved facilities and better equipment have also played their part in raising performance standards. This is evidenced by comparing Olympic records of past years with those of the present day. In some events, Olympic gold medal winners of the early 1900s would probably not even qualify to compete in today's finals.

One of the reasons for the international upsurge of interest in sport is the greater availability of leisure time in today's world. This has had the effect of stimulating people to look for ways of filling their time, either by watching or participating in sport. The wide coverage of sport on television has also contributed to this explosion of interest. Inevitably, it is the performances of the best competitors, the elite sportspeople, which attract the most attention. Their successes gain national and international prestige: those who win in international sport bring great kudos to their country. In addition, their performance successes act as models for those of us who are less gifted. Thus every weekend golfer would like to hit the ball like Greg Norman and social tennis players long for the finesse and power of Ivan Lendl. This desire to model our sporting behaviours on those of our sporting heroes is commendable, providing we realise that we probably do not possess their natural skills or flair.

What determines success?

Whether you are an elite athlete (using the term 'athlete' in the broad generic sense of anyone who participates in sport), or just play sport as a leisure activity, there are certain fundamentals that will determine your success. These are your innate or inborn talent for that sport, the amount of coaching and practice you have, and your psychological approach to the game.

The psychological component

The way you approach sport psychologically can have a most significant bearing on how well you perform, especially in competition. If you have any doubts about this, compare your performance when you are 'hitting up' in a friendly tennis game or playing a practice round of golf, with how you react in a serious match. The stress of competition seems to cast quite a different light on how you play. Generally when you try a little harder this causes you to imperceptibly 'tighten up', so that you play shots quite differently from the way you did in the practice situation. In a sense, you have 'choked' under pressure, and this stems from mental stress.

Walking the mental plank

No one is immune to this competition stress. The weekend

golfer waiting to hit off the first tee in a club event is just as likely to be affected as the elite athlete participating in an international event. You can get a feel for this by noting the words of Kim Hughes, the former Australian cricket captain, following his team's defeat in a test match against England in 1981. In a newspaper interview he said 'Cricket is so much of a mental thing and a player who is brilliant in the nets can freeze in the middle. You lay a plank on the ground and ask someone to walk across it—no problem. Suspend the plank between two rooftops and . . . that's what crept in.'

Helping sportspeople walk this 'mental plank' has resulted in the development of a new branch of psychology—sports psychology. Many of the leading sporting bodies in countries such as the USA, USSR, Sweden, Japan and in the Eastern Bloc have long recognised the importance of the mental factor in sport. They have accepted that, irrespective of talent and specialised training, unless an athlete is correctly prepared from a psychological point of view, he or she will not perform to potential in the heat of international competition.[48] Along with this goes the recognition that competition stress is not confined to selected sports but occurs across a wide spectrum.[49]

Your major opponent

If you are to beat this sports bogey, the first thing you have to accept is that your major opponent is often *yourself* and, as with many things in life, recognising the problem is halfway to treating it. The second step is to identify the ways in which competition stress affects you and your performance.

Tension in your body

Although it is helpful to differentiate between physical and mental stress, you should understand that muscle tension arises because the mind is overloaded and finding it hard to cope. In other words, if you are relaxed in your mind then you will be relaxed in your body. However, body tension is not always easy to recognise. In sports involving your holding a ball, bat, racquet, club or rifle, even the smallest amount of tension in your hands or fingers will interfere with your sense of control.

The first parts of the body usually affected by stress are the fingers, hands and forearms. You only need to tighten your grip a little on a ball, bat, club or racquet for you to lose speed, direction, swing or power. This can also contribute to the loss of 'feel' that many sportspeople comment upon.

The importance of a relaxed grip just cannot be overemphasised. Greg Norman uses the term 'pressure' to describe tension in the hands:

> *Most people I see playing golf get on the*
> *first tee and the pressure in their hands*
> *gets very tense. You can see the whites of*
> *their knuckles coming out because they*
> *are tight: they are tense and nervous . . .*
> *I'm a strong believer when you grip the*
> *golf club, if someone came along they*
> *could pull it out of your hands.*[50]

But sportspeople do not experience tension solely in the hands and arms. Tension in the neck, back, shoulders and legs is a common experience and is part of the general 'tightening up' that happens when you are stressed.

How tension affects performance

The principal effect of tension in any of the body muscles is to interfere with rhythm, balance and timing. Your coordination becomes impaired and there is a general loss of ease in all the actions associated with your sport. Fine judgement is lost, perhaps due to loss of that intangible factor called 'feel'. In certain sports this may not be an important factor, but in others, such as rifle and pistol shooting, it can be critical.

Another tension effect in athletes, and one that should not be overlooked, is the danger of muscle injury. Muscles free from tension contract and relax in response to the demands placed upon them. On the other hand, muscle tension or 'being physically uptight' can lead to muscle spasm. When you place an extra strain on these muscles, as in exercise, there is a very real possibility of tearing some of the muscle fibres. This causes bleeding into the muscles (known as a haematoma), and leads to pain and difficulty in movement.

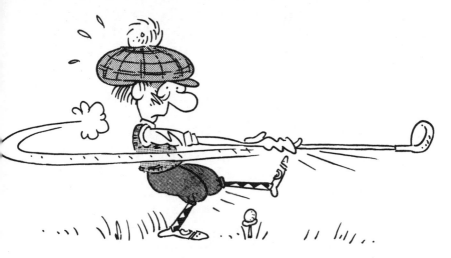

Muscle tension interferes with rhythm, balance and
timing

What you have to realise is that stretching exercises carried
out before a competitive event may not, in themselves, produce
sufficient muscle relaxation if the mind is still tense. If, on
the other hand, you are relaxed in your mind, you are far less
likely to sustain injury.

A third effect of muscle tension is that it wastes energy, and
this can be crucial for athletes who perform in endurance events.
Learning to relax in your sport, therefore, will improve your
endurance by helping your body use up oxygen and stored
kilojoules in the most efficient way.[51]

The mental factor

Have you ever wondered why there are days when you perform
with ease in your sport, and others when everything seems
so much effort and you appear to have little 'touch' in your
play? The answer lies in how you feel mentally on the day.
Although this is not of serious consquence to most of us, for
professional sportspeople it can be a matter of some concern.
Their livelihood usually depends on consistency of performance
and it is therefore little wonder that they go to considerable
lengths to control these mental factors.

Anyone, whether involved at an amateur or professional level, can experience performance stress. When it occurs, not only does it undermine how well you function but it also interferes with that most important factor—your sense of enjoyment. To some extent, *you* become your own worst enemy. Once you master your own stress problems you are in much better shape to cope with an opponent.

Your arousal: too much or too little

There would be few people who participate in sport familiar with the term arousal, for it is not a word commonly used in sport. In the psychological world it refers to the degree of energy release, or the readiness to react to varying situations. Most athletes aim to achieve a high level of arousal by becoming 'psyched up' or 'getting the adrenaline flowing', believing that this will ensure a better performance, but is this necessarily the case?

The answer to this question is not a straightforward one and depends on the type of sport or, in a team game, the role that a player has to take. Body contact sports, for example, would call for a higher level of arousal than, say, tennis, golf or rifle shooting. In general terms, however, there is an optimal level of arousal, and if this is exceeded performance tends to decline. This view was first proposed in 1908 by Yerkes and Dodson, who suggested that too low or too high arousal interfered with performance and the aim should be to achieve an ideal level. They depicted this in the form of an inverted-u graph:

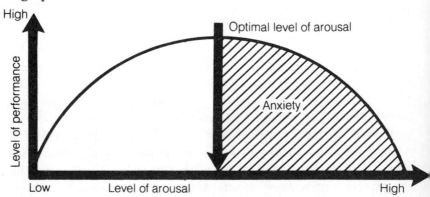

Once your level of arousal becomes excessive you enter the realm of stress or anxiety. In order for you to play to your best ability you must therefore first be able to monitor your body for tell-tale signs of stress, and secondly, have ways of reducing this if and when required. As we will see later, self-hypnosis and the use of relaxation cues will enable you to do this.

The effects of arousal on your attention

We are all aware of the need to be able to concentrate on the ball if we are catching it, or on an opponent if we are are going to tackle or block his progress. Failure to achieve or maintain attentional focusing (another term for concentration) can lead to our dropping the ball or missing the tackle. Although we may admit that we 'lost concentration' at the critical moment, it is important to have some understanding as to the underlying cause if we wish to avoid repeating the error. And so we return to arousal, for if it is too high it interferes with fine muscle movements, coordination, steadiness and, above all, concentration.

The varieties of concentration

Attentional focusing or concentration is a complex issue. You utilise different types of focusing depending on the type of sport you play and the immediate needs of the moment. In general terms, you have an external type, which is involved in being aware of changing conditions around you, and an internal one which monitors your thoughts, feelings and ideas. To complicate things still further, each of these types has two widths—a broad and a narrow[52] somewhat like a wide-angle and a close-up lens on a camera.

Your external mental lenses

Whenever you participate in your sport, the chances are that you are constantly changing your focus of attention (or mental lens) from broad to narrow to broad without even realising it. Thus a golfer may, at one moment, be called upon to assess the slope of the fairway, the position of hazards or the wind direction (broad external). On reaching the putting green, the mental lens has to change (narrow external) in order to determine the correct line for the putt, and the slope and pace of the green. Having completed putting, the focus automatically returns to becoming broad once again.

Stress and your external focusing

But what happens if you are stressed? This usually results in your being unable to shift your focus to that of being a close-up lens. You become easily distracted by things around you— other players, extraneous noise, even leaves blowing across the green. The result is that you fail to give your full attention to the task in hand and make a bad putt.

Sometimes excessive arousal can have the reverse effect and narrow your attention too much so that you are unable to change to your wide-angle lens when required. Golfers sometimes relate that, when playing exceptionally well and above their normal standards, they become tired and 'lose momentum' over the closing stages of the match. What has happened is that their excessive arousal has led to a persistent narrowing of their concentration focus. Because this 'adrenaline effect' is tiring if it continues for too long, in time it leads to a decreased performance. These effects of excessive arousal are, of course, relevant to most sports.

Your internal mental lenses

Just as there are two external foci of concentration, so too are there two internal ones.[52] You employ your narrow internal focus when you are mentally rehearsing and preparing for a game. This type of mental focusing is particularly helpful in golf, shooting and distance running, where you need to concentrate on one stimulus at a time. Good distance runners, for example, are able to distract their mind from painful feelings by focusing on their running style and rhythm. In this case, the use of the internal mental lens has the effect of increasing their pain tolerance.

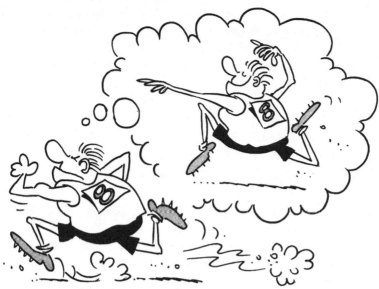

Marathon runners focus on style and rhythm to
overcome pain

Your broad internal mental lens tends to come into operation when you are reflecting on a game, planning the way you are going to play it and how you will counter particular moves that an opponent may make. In this reflective state, you will often analyse past mistakes so that you can ensure you will deal with similar situations in the future in a more positive way.

The techniques used by Peter T. provide a wonderful example of how you can use your broad, internal focusing. Peter is a paraplegic, and a champion performer in wheelchair athletics. At various stages he has held the world record in wheelchair events for 400, 1500 and 10 000 metre distances. He had been a regular competitor in the Paralympics, where he won the gold medal in the 5000 metre event in 1984. Occasionally he competes in marathons, but enters these 'only for the fun of it' and as a way of improving his endurance capacity.

He describes the way in which he uses his broad internal mental lens in this way: 'I imagine myself lining up at the start with other competitors. After I have gone 100 metres, I think "Where am I; where do I want to be?" Sometimes as a way of motivating myself, I imagine a major competitor 20 metres ahead of me and going hard. I have to catch him. The harder he pushes, the harder I push until I catch him.'

Peter finds this use of his broad internal focus of attention (mental rehearsal) a very necessary part of his preparation for any major event. His approach is typical of a great many sportspeople, both professional and amateur. It indicates the important role that correct mental preparation can have on your sporting performance.

Stress and internal focusing

Stress unquestionably makes a difference to your inner mental focusing, even if you are not aware of it. A study done on swimmers has demonstrated that when they are stressed they perform inconsistently and poorly.[52] Just as you need to be able to smoothly change your external lenses in keeping with the changing demands of the situation, so too must you be able to move your internal one from broad to narrow and back again. Stress tends to interfere with your ability to interchange your mental foci of attention.

What happens to stressed performers in swimming is that they tend to narrow their attentional focus too much and have difficulty in opening it up again. Because they lose their wide-angle view of things, they fail to take in what is happening around them and are unable to make changes in strategy to meet the needs of the moment. This may result in their 'choking' under the pressure of competition. Often they let past mistakes disrupt subsequent performance and, unlike Peter T., have difficulty planning ahead about how they are going to cope with a variety of possible scenarios.

This raises another important issue with regard to the correct use of your broad inner mental lens. When you use this technique it is necessary to imagine yourself having to cope satisfactorily with a variety of possible situations. If you are a track athlete, for example, you should visualise how you will respond (a) if you are leading as you come into the final straight, (b) if you have someone running hard alongside you, and (c) if you are being overtaken in the last 100 metres of the race. Unless you have prepared your mind for all these possibilities, it is unreasonable to expect it to react as you would wish when something unexpected occurs during an actual race.

Your expectation to do well

Anyone who plays sport is aware of how important it is to feel confident. When we talk of confidence we are usually referring to our having a belief in ourselves—a belief that we can perform well, improve our standards and perhaps win the particular event in which we are competing. But confidence, or, to be more accurate, self-esteem, is a fragile psychological factor. It can be undermined by seemingly small changes in fortune. Even a chance remark from an opponent can be sufficient to set in motion a whole series of events which can dent your self-esteem. It is a tactic which is often deliberately employed by competitors to 'psyche out' the opposition.

Relaxed sportspeople who have taken the trouble to mentally prepare for competition are rarely subject to the problems of low self-worth. They go into events with an expectation that they can do well, play their shots or do whatever is called for in their sport. The aim is to see yourself winning. This was nicely summed up by Peter T. when he said 'The most important part of the mental rehearsal is seeing yourself winning. You have to see yourself beating other people: the look of disappointment on their face and the look of exhilaration on yours.'

Losing self-esteem

Stress is unquestionably the most potent factor in causing you to lose self-esteem. Competitors often attribute confidence loss to their having experienced a series of failures or 'outs' in their sport. What many fail to realise is that the problem arose initially because of tension or stress. In an effort to break the pattern of failures they consciously 'try' even harder to do well, and this then leads to even more stress and tension. The cycle is best depicted as:

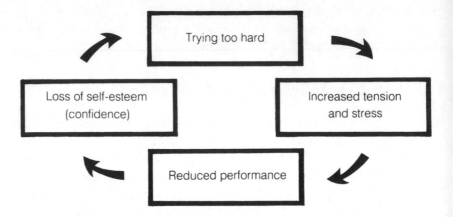

As you will see later, the aim will be to break this cycle by achieving relaxation and unconscious re-programming of the mind through self-hypnosis.

Fears in sport

Fear is a not uncommon experience for many sports participants. The most frequent fear that competitors have to face is a fear of failure and it occurs whether we play sport purely at a social or at an international level.

Fear of failure

No one likes to do badly and this could be one reason for fearing failure. Another is tied in with our concern as to how others perceive our performance. In other words, it is closely related to self-esteem and self-perception, for not only is it necessary for us to do well but also to be seen to have done so by others.

Those who have the skills and talent to perform at higher levels of competition, especially in national or international events, are more likely to be subjected to the sorts of pressures that lead to fear of failure. They are often in the limelight and their performances are constantly being scrutinised by the media, team colleagues, coaches and the public at large. It is not surprising, therefore, that these athletes become stressed in major events, that is, unless they have developed the mental skills to cope with such situations.

Fear of injury

Another fear that can trouble any sports competitor is the fear of injury. A behaviour inherent in you is that of self-preservation. If something is likely to harm you, your natural inclination is to avoid it, or take steps to protect yourself from it. This avoidance behaviour is reinforced if you have suffered injury of some kind in a similar situation in the past. In effect, you become fearful of that situation. Even though this fear may not be at a conscious level, it will still affect the way you respond and may interfere with your willingness to confront that particular sports situation again. This was exemplified by Ann P., an eighteen-year-old diver. She was considered to have great potential and had won many major diving events, including state titles at various board heights. In practising a new and complex manoeuvre from the high board, she failed to complete the turns and landed face-downwards on the water. This had the effect of hurting not only her body but also her self-esteem. As a result, she felt unable to attempt this particular dive again and was even reluctant to try any other dives from the 10 metre board.

Treatment in hypnosis and self-hypnosis was directed at desensitising her from her fear through the use of imagery. She was able to reestablish her confidence in her ability to dive from the high board, and finally was able to perform the dive which she feared in a very satisfactory way.

Fear arising from injury can also affect style. Some sort of mental protective device within us inhibits our being able to carry out an action which, previously, was second nature to us. Consider the case of Marie J. who broke a bone in her left foot whilst competing in the 100 metre hurdle event at an international event. When she returned to running and hurdling after her injury, she found that she was unable to 'snap' her leading foot firmly downwards as she cleared each hurdle. This led to her changing her style and, not surprisingly, led to poor performances and a loss of form.

She was aware that the injury had created a fear of a similar thing happening again. Therapy in hypnosis and self-hypnosis was directed towards breaking down the fear and restoring confidence in her ability to hurdle as in the past. She used a great deal of imagery in self-hypnosis to restore her previous style, and subsequently competed with success.

COPING WITH SPORTS PROBLEMS

As I have shown, stress can have the most damaging of effects on your performance. Using self-hypnosis on a regular, daily basis will provide you with a method of breaking down the stresses in your mind and body. On its own it can provide the necessary relaxation which will enable your mind and body to function efficiently, whatever your sporting endeavour. As you will see later, when it is linked with suggestion or imagery, it will enable you to work upon and change other patterns of behaviour which bother you.

Your relaxation cue

Sometimes tension and stress can come 'out of the blue' when you are faced by a competition situation, or a vital point in the match when pressures are starting to build. At these times it is important for you to have a cue or mechanism which will immediately reduce the stress and help to restore your mental equilibrium.

The cue which may prove helpful to you is one which you already utilise in the induction of your self-hypnosis. It entails thinking of the word 'calm' every time you breathe out, until you feel a sense of calmness and relaxation in your body and mind. For this cue to become effective, it will need constant reinforcement, preferably at times when you are not particularly stressed. Thus, you should practice it each day for fifteen to twenty seconds as often as you can remember to do so. The more you reinforce it, the more powerful and involuntary it will become, so that when you are under pressure your mind will call upon the cue to bring your stress down to levels where you feel comfortable.

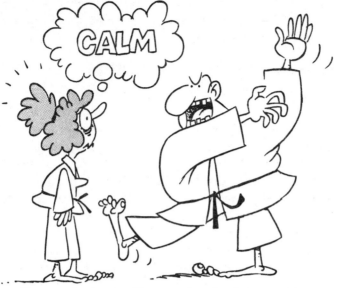

You can 'cue' yourself to remain calm in competition situations

Improving your confidence

Belief in yourself is a most important prerequisite if you want to do well in your sport. Imagine, for example, you are playing your weekend round of golf. You may be worried about whether you are going to hit a particular shot out of bounds, and curiously the very thing you fear happening actually occurs. It is almost as though you have no control over it.

This occurs because your fear of doing something wrong has undermined your confidence in hitting the ball normally. It is worthwhile reminding yourself from time to time of the intense power of the unconscious mind. If stress creeps in, it can soon have a significant effect on your self-belief and affect the way your body functions. Without necessarily being aware of it, you will tighten up in the muscles of your hands, arms and back and this will lead to all sorts of peculiarities in your swing.

If your self-belief is influenced so strongly by stress, your first aim is obviously to develop a relaxed approach to your game. In spite of advice, often given gratuitiously, it is simply not possible to *try* to relax. Any conscious striving to relax will either have no effect at all or will create even more tension. This is why the re-programming of your unconscious mind through self-hypnosis can be so beneficial.

Restructuring your thoughts

In self-hypnosis your mind is extremely sensitive to suggestions and imagery, and it makes good sense, therefore, to use this facility in order to change the things you want to change. Before you start, it is necessary to decide what suggestions you are going to silently give yourself. This is where your work diary (see Chapter 4) can be of help. The notes you take will enable you to recognise problem areas in your game so that you can then write down and memorise those suggestions which will enable you to counteract them. Although this may seem burdensome at first, remember that you are going to use many of the same suggestions each time you use self-hypnosis. Hence the initial effort is well worthwhile. (Although golf is being used as our model, the same principles apply no matter what your sport.)

Suggestions must always be couched in positive terms. All too often people, without realising it, inculcate negative thoughts such as 'I am *not* going to move my head when I hit the ball'. The following suggestions may give you a flavour of the things you should say to yourself in self-hypnosis:

> *Whenever I play . . . I am going to*
> *enjoy my game . . . and play each shot in*
> *a relaxed way. I will feel the relaxation in*
> *my fingers . . . in my hands . . . in my*
> *arms and shoulders so that when I swing*
> *the club . . . I can feel the weight of the*
> *club head throughout. Because my mind*
> *will feel calm and at ease . . . I will be*
> *able to swing in a relaxed, effortless way*
> *. . . hitting the ball just as I want to.*
>
> *As I set up for each shot . . . I will find*
> *it so easy to get a mental picture of where*
> *I want it to go . . . and the way to play it.*

I can use my relaxation cue . . . as I walk
around the course. This will help me relax
even more . . . and remind me to use my
mental imagery . . . with every shot that I
play.

These suggestions are of a general nature, and you may wish to incorporate others that are more specifically related to some aspect of your game. The aim is to restructure your thoughts so that they operate in a way, and at the time, that you want them to. This unconscious processing will help rebuild your self-esteem to the point where you expect to play well.

You may have noticed in the sample suggestions above that reference is made to your use of mental imagery. Whatever your sport, visualising correct responses in self-hypnosis will go a long way towards ensuring that these behaviours occur. They will lead to your mentally anticipating that you are going to perform in the correct way.

Visualisation can certainly improve performance. It can do this in several ways: by goal programming (showing the body what to do), through learning (getting the body accustomed to how to do it), and by increasing confidence in your abilities. This was demonstrated in a Swedish study carried out on basketball players.[53] Subjects were divided into three groups: the first practiced thirty free throws a day for two weeks, the second mentally rehearsed these throws but did not physically practice, and the third did neither. When tested at the end of the period of study, the players who had only mentally rehearsed the throws achieved the same results as those who had physically practised. The control group ran a poor third. If mental rehearsal can be so effective when used on its own, you can well imagine how powerful a tool it becomes when incorporated into a relaxed state such as self-hypnosis.

Your powers of concentration

From our earliest days at school we were told of the importance of concentration, but rarely were we shown how to concentrate correctly. It comes as no surprise therefore, to find that few of us can focus our concentration or attention as we would like when we play sport.

The relaxation afforded by self-hypnosis is extremely helpful in the focusing of attention, and it also has the advantage of providing you with a means to train your mind so that you can change your mental lenses from broad to narrow, or vice versa, whenever you wish.

Using imagery in self-hypnosis is probably the best way to teach your mind to smoothly change focus. In swimming, for example, if you narrow down your mental focus too much, you will fail to 'take in' what other swimmers are doing around you. If that happens, it requires little knowledge of swimming to know what the outcome will be. Similarly in golf you need to be able to change from a wide-angle external lens when you are walking along a fairway, to a narrow one when confronted by a putt.

In your mentally disengaged state of self-hypnosis, picture yourself, for example, walking along a fairway at your own course. See yourself focusing on a variety of things around you— the position of hazards, the wind direction, the position of the pin on the putting green. These factors will determine how you play your next shot. Next, imagine yourself on the putting green, only now you have changed to your narrow external lens and the only things you see are those relevant to the line along which you are going to putt. Rather than visualise a line, you will probably find it easier to picture the ball going along a track or pathway to the hole. You can make this as wide as you wish but it should rarely be wider than the diameter of the hole itself.

Mentally practising changing your focus of attention will soon ensure that the process happens automatically on the course. The more you practise this imagery, the easier it will be to integrate it into your everyday game. This aspect was rather nicely expressed by Patmore when she wrote: 'Images are better than words, it seems, because they can over-ride intellectual difficulties. The image must be stamped clearly and repeatedly, and in as much detail as possible. This is the way in which the body receives its instructions. A whole series of movements which the body is required to perform can be inculcated in this way, providing the instructions are given clearly and confidently.'[49]

In any sport you can teach your mind to focus intensely on something or to open up so that you become aware of peripheral things. Both of these concentration processes are necessary if you wish to perform well.

How to cope with fear

Earlier it was suggested that people who play sport can face two types of fear: fear of failure and fear of injury. Both types can be treated in similar ways using self-hypnosis. The main thrust of treatment must be directed towards having the person eventually 'see' themselves performing well and without fear. This can be done by using imagery. Known as imaginal desensitisation, this process involves the person visualising themselves, whilst in self-hypnosis, learning to cope with a number of scenes associated with their fears.

In order to understand the rationale behind this, imagine a future event in your sport in which you would like to do well. But suppose you performed badly in a similar event in the past. The chances are that you would have a certain amount of trepidation about how you are going to respond on the day. You might be concerned about letting down other team members or by what others may think if you repeat your bad performances. The seeds of fear of failure have been sown and are already germinating.

Where this is the case, the first step is to recognise how damaging this fear can be to your performance. For serious sportspeople it can be an issue of tremendous importance. Once you have come to terms with the fact that it is bothering you, you can set about correcting it.

In your work diary, write down a hierarchy of scenes which you are going to visualise in self-hypnosis. Start with a scene distant from the feared occasion and therefore the least fearful. Follow with scenes which bring you closer to the event until the final one is of you actually competing. Here are some sample hierarchy scenes:

1. It is the day before the event and you are at home with your family. You are thinking about the competition tomorrow.
2. It is the morning of the event. You are at home, surrounded by people and things familiar to you.
3. You are in your car driving to the place where you are going to perform.
4. You arrive at the ground and you are making your way to the changing room.
5. You walk outside and see a large crowd of people. Some of these you know. Most are unfamiliar to you.
6. You are waiting for your turn to compete. It seems a long time. You are aware of the noise of the crowd.
7. Your competition time has arrived. You realise that many people are watching every move you make.

Having written down the scenes in increasing order of fear, the next step is to set up your own fear meter. You could view this as being like a thermometer, measuring your fear levels on a scale of 0 to 100.

It is helpful to accurately measure how much fear you feel in a particular scene rather than depend on vague assessments such as 'a little bit' or 'a great deal'. You will find that your mind has the capacity to estimate your level of fear. If this is 50 or over on your scale, you can consider it to be too high.

Imagining the feared scene

In self-hypnosis, visualise the first scene in your hierarchy in as much detail as possible. Picture the furniture in your home and the view you can see from the window. If you have had a similar experience in the past, remember it, imagine it, and experience that scene again.[54] Once you are able to re-experience yourself in that scene with vivid intensity, turn your attention to your fear meter and assess how fearful you are. If the fear level is high, you may also notice physical symptoms such as a rapid heart rate, sweating or tremulousness. You should not be too concerned by these for although they are unpleasant, they will prove to be transient and indicate how involved you are in your fear situation.

Using your mental haven

If the level is over 50 on your scale, take a break from the fear situation for a while and let your mind take you into another scene. You may wish to go into your own inner mental place. Imagine you are walking along a beautiful corridor in your mind until you come to a door. When you open it and step inside, you find yourself in a tranquil place—one in which nothing and no one can harm or disturb you in any way. As you close the door behind you, you shut out all negative feelings, including your fears. Spend as long as you wish exploring that special place in your mind, quite free from concerns and worries.

Once you are entirely at ease and feel ready to confront the fear situation again, visualise yourself leaving your peaceful place, closing the door behind you and retracing your steps along your mind's corridor. When you return to the sports scene you will probably find that the fear levels are not nearly as high as before. But if they are still above 50 on your scale, go back to that special place in your mind where you felt so much peace.

You should continue to alternate between these two scenes until your fear reduces to a level where you feel comfortable. This will probably be in the region of 25 to 30 on your scale: it is impracticable for you to try and attain a zero reading.

Once you have conquered your fear in one scene, you can then move on to the next one in your hierarchy and repeat the procedure. You may find it takes many sessions of this desensitisation process before you finally visualise and conquer the fear in your competition scene. In order to reinforce the gains you have achieved, you should end by imagining yourself competing successfully and with a sense of enjoyment.

This self-hypnotic visualisation technique allows you to confront and deal with things you may fear in a sporting situation and does so by introducing you to them in a gradual way. It allows you to proceed at your own pace and you have the advantage of being able to choose when you feel ready and comfortable to move on to the next scene. Your goal is to feel at ease in the real life situation, and this imaginal procedure will certainly help you achieve this.

CHAPTER SEVEN

MIND CONTROL OVER YOUR PAIN

When you hit your thumb with a hammer or put your hand on the hotplate of an electric stove, your first impression is one of pain. This sets up a reflex action designed to protect you from further damage, and so you drop the hammer or withdraw your hand. What we are talking about here is short-duration or acute pain. Little more need be said about this, since it will usually settle on its own with symptomatic treatment such as ice, aspirin or your favoured remedy.

Chronic or long-term pain, on the other hand, poses quite a different set of problems altogether. By convention, it is classed as being chronic when it has been present for at least six months, and differs from the acute variety by generally becoming worse with time. For the person who suffers from chronic pain, one off the hardest things to bear is the fact that treatment usually produces temporary relief only, the symptoms reappearing after a short while.

Not surprisingly, this leads many patients to try out a wide variety of therapeutic approaches in a desperate bid to minimise their suffering. It is certainly true that what seems to work for one person does not necessarily work for another, and a natural consequence of this is that many hospitals throughout the world have set up pain clinics (perhaps pain-*relief* clinics would be a more apt term). These are staffed by doctors from a number of medical disciplines—anaesthetists, neurologists, acupuncturists, hypnotherapists and surgeons—who offer treatment in their own particular field of expertise.

Problems associated with chronic pain

Why has there been a greater interest in the treatment of chronic pain in recent years? Chronic pain can be one of the most disabling and distressing of symptoms, and it is undoubtedly one of the hardest to treat successfully. Its effects are far-ranging, sometimes being so incapacitating that work becomes impossible. Not only does this have a seriously damaging effect on the morale of the sufferer but also, as one would expect, on the whole family constellation. Money often becomes scarce and frequently the spouse has to work to supplement sickness benefits as well as maintain the home. Because the pain sufferer has difficulty in getting about, social activities tend to become restricted or non-existent. To add to the patient's tale of woe, the ever-present pain may impede or make sexual intercourse impossible. Clearly, it is a disorder which can wreak havoc in even the most stable of families.

Then there is the financial effect on the community at large. Diseases which cause chronic pain have been shown to have a major impact on the nation's economy. Arthritis is a good example of this. A study carried out in Australia in 1981[55] reported that arthritis is the most frequently reported chronic condition of ill health, affecting 1.1 million, or 8 per cent of the population. It was estimated that lost earnings due to arthritis amounted to approximately $300 million each year. To underline the magnitude of the problem still further, 5.2 million working days were lost due to arthritis in 1981—25 per cent more than the total number of working days lost due to all industrial disputes that year. In other countries the incidence seems to be even higher. A National Health Interview Survey conducted in the USA in 1979 revealed that 120 per 1000 of the population suffered from arthritis. These statistics are frightening and indicate how common the problem of chronic pain really is.

The nature of pain

If you are unfortunate enough to suffer from chronic pain, you could be forgiven for wondering why, in these days of more enlightened medical treatment, something cannot be done to ease your burden. It may not be of much solace to you, but it is not for the want of trying. Physicians throughout the world are constantly seeking new ways of breaking the pain syndrome, but the problem continues to march on inexorably.

The main difficulty stems from our inability to assess what pain actually is. This may seem curious, but you have to realise that although your pain is very real and distressing to you, it is a symptom and not a physical sign. While you may describe it as stabbing, gripping or burning in nature, these are not things which can be seen or measured like a fever. You are the only one who *feels* that pain. There is no instrument known to man which can measure its intensity.

Admittedly, we can measure the *effects* that pain can sometimes have on the body by assessing heart rate, blood pressure or brain tracings (electroencephalograms), but these are indirect measurements and do not always indicate to what degree you are suffering. It is to suffering that I will constantly allude, for that is the only word that truly describes what the chronic pain patient experiences.

How you feel pain in your brain

Although most of us refer to pain as a sensation, this is not an accurate term. Sensation is associated with seeing, hearing, touching and the movements in our muscles and joints. But if it is not a sensation, what is it? To get some idea of this, let us return to the situation where you hit your thumb with a hammer. You will say that you have a pain in your thumb, but in fact the pain is situated in your brain. When the hammer struck your thumb, a series of messages passed through the nerves in your hand and arm to your brain, where they were interpreted as pain by special nerve cells.

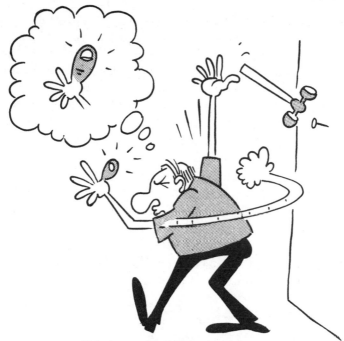

Pain is actually 'felt' in the brain

All of this may explain the physiology of pain but it still does not tell us what it really is. The Greek philosopher Aristotle was very close to an explanation when he suggested that pain is an emotion. It is now recognised that there is a very strong emotional component to chronic pain. As we will see later, it is often associated with marked feelings of anxiety (stress) and depression. This is not to suggest that the pain experience is in any way imaginary, for nothing could be further from the truth. If, for example, you suffer chronic low back pain because of pressure on certain nerves as they issue from your spinal canal, the symptoms you feel are very real and are caused by the irritation of these nerves. However, as in the example of the damaged thumb, you may *feel* the pain in your back or legs but it is your brain cells which are the main culprits.

The gate control mechanism

How can we be so sure that pain is really in the brain? Perhaps the most widely accepted explanation to support this view is the 'gate control theory'.[56] Put simply, it proposes that in a certain part of the brain there is a mechanism that acts as a pain gate. This area is supplied by two types of nerves, one having a large and the other a small diameter. The large ones carry messages which partially close the gate and thus help block the pain. This pain blockade is not a total one because pain has a vital role in alerting you to damage somewhere in your body. The small diameter nerves have the opposite effect, and by opening the gate, allow pain messages to get through to the brain.

Whenever you become stressed, anxious or worried, this acts to stimulate the small fibres, and because this has the effect of opening the gate, it causes you to feel more pain. When you are relaxed, on the other hand, these messages pass up the large nerve fibres, close the gate and reduce the pain experience. And so you can see the need for you to relax is not a fanciful notion.

The purpose of pain

Pain is there to tell you (and others) that *something is wrong*. Your brain does this by sending signals back to the original site of hurt to point out that some damage, irritation or inflammation has occurred. It does this so that you will take appropriate action to deal with the cause.

Thus, if you hit your thumb with a hammer, your immediate reaction is to drop the hammer and remove your thumb. In the case of chronic pain, you take steps to find out and treat whatever it is that creates your discomfort. How you react to the pain experience thereafter is very much tied to your emotional state. Unless you give some thought to how your mind is responding to the messages it receives, and deal with the situation, you may find that the pain will continue to bother you, perhaps becoming more intense. Once you accept the principle of dealing with the mind aspect of pain, however, you are well on the way to easing your distress.

Effects on your emotional state

All of us have suffered pain at some stage or other, and when we have we may have been aware that it caused us to feel tense, upset and worried. In other words, it caused us to feel stressed or anxious. In the case of acute pain, these feelings tend to be short-lived and self-limiting, but for people who are chronic sufferers the position becomes far more complex.

One of the first effects of pain is that it causes an increase in muscle tension, not only near the site of damage but generally throughout the body, and this tends to further intensify the symptom.[57] A vicious cycle of pain $\longrightarrow$ muscle tension $\longrightarrow$ increased pain is soon established which, even for the most stoic of people, can prove hard to bear.

With time, chronic pain produces effects on personality. Feelings of helplessness and despair soon emerge and may be accompanied by irritability and loss of interest in everyday things. Sleep becomes impaired and the sufferer experiences a constant sense of fatigue. There is often an erosion of personal relationships with family and friends, and loss of sexual interest can add greatly to marital strain.

It requires no great knowledge of the workings of the human mind to realise at this stage that the pain is now creating great stress and even depression in that person. The factor that is affected *most of all* by this distressing condition is self-esteem, patients who have been in pain for a long time often describing their confidence and self-worth as 'zilch'. Once this vital personality factor becomes undermined, it inevitably leads to a loss of will to fight the disorder or to become involved in anything worthwhile.

The complex interplay between stress, pain and various psychological factors can best be illustrated by this flow chart:

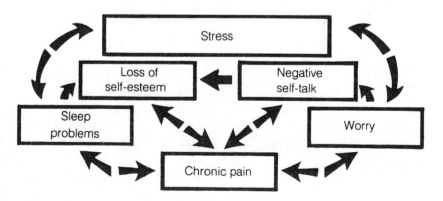

Protecting yourself from pain

If pain has troubled you for a long while, the chances are that there are occasions when you feel that you are never going to be able to get on top of it. Your feelings of helplessness and defencelessness are not unlike those you would experience if you were shut in a cage with a savage animal and without any means of protection. In addition, the negative effects of stress that would arise in such a situation would make you less likely to devise ways of preventing being attacked.

Self-hypnotic techniques will enable you to confront this savage animal (the pain) knowing that you *do* have ways of protecting yourself. This can prove very reassuring and comforting, especially as these procedures are always readily available: you carry them with you in your mind wherever you go and whatever you do. It only needs practice on a regular basis for them to become powerful and effective. Keep reminding yourself of one thing: if the mind can play such a major role in creating and intensifying your pain, then it can also be controlled to diminish that experience. You are the coach and how you train your mind to use pain-coping strategies will determine how successful it will be.

The denial factor

There is one piece of folklore that seems to have been handed down from person to person over many generations. It is the belief that if you are suffering pain you should not talk about it or focus on it for fear of making it worse. Believing in this notion is tantamount to saying 'if we don't think about it, it will go away'. This makes no more sense than believing that if you are feverish, your temperature will drop if you ignore it.

This denial approach probably arose because, in years gone by, people had few ways of dealing with suffering. This is no longer true and the idea you must firmly establish in your mind at the outset is that pain need not be an unchanging experience. You *can* do a great deal to help yourself diminish its effects.

Before you embark on your self-control techniques, two other points need to be emphasised. Whatever the source of your pain, it is mandatory for you to seek medical treatment for it. Your pain indicates that something is wrong, so it makes good sense to determine what that something is before you start dealing with the mind factors.

The need for realistic expectations

Many people start into self-therapy with the belief that they are going to remove their pain completely. When this fails to happen they become discouraged and abandon self-hypnosis, considering it to be valueless for them. The problem here lies not in self-hypnosis being ineffective but in the person having unrealistic expectations.

The aim in treating chronic pain with self-hypnosis is to *ease* the symptom by changing your perception of it. Rarely, if ever, does one set out to obliterate it. In any case, this could prove dangerous for it would remove one of the ways the body has for telling you all is not well yet in the damaged area. Once you accept this idea, and set out on the treatment path with realistic goals, you will find self-hypnosis to be a useful ally.

Removing negative barriers

Some people enter into treatment without enthusiasm, anticipating from the start that they are going to gain little benefit from it. This fear of failure is almost certainly born of stress and depression. The problem is of some magnitude: in an Australian health survey carried out in 1977–78, 22 per cent of patients suffering from arthritis did not consult their doctor because they felt they could not be helped.[55]

Even if your pain is severe and intractable you *can* do a great deal towards diminishing it. You will need patience and perseverance in using the self-hypnotic techniques, but you will be rewarded by a noticeable improvement in your mental state, and the comfort of knowing that you have the pain under *your* control, instead of the other way round.

Pain, by its very nature, is associated with a host of other symptoms. Tension, irritability, feelings of helplessness and insomnia are but a few of the many that form the chronic pain syndrome. Becoming aware that these are part of the overall pain picture is the first essential step.

The value of your work diary

You may not find it easy, at first, to accept that your psychological and bodily symptoms are related to pain. This is where your work diary can be of immense value. By keeping a daily record of the pain occurrences, their intensity and nature, and the way you feel emotionally at these times, will soon give you considerable insight. Having come to terms with the interrelationship between pain and your stress problems, you will be in a better position to do something constructive about letting them go.

TREATING YOUR PAIN EXPERIENCE

The effects of relaxation

Over the years, many studies have shown that relaxation can be of considerable benefit in reducing pain.[58] Given this to be the case, you may question why you should go to the trouble of learning and practising a more involved procedure like self-hypnosis. When we consider relaxation techniques, we usually think of them in terms of their physical effects on the body, perhaps describing the body as feeling floppy and loose. Although there is an associated state of mental ease when you use simple relaxation procedures, this is not present to any marked degree.

Self-hypnosis, on the other hand, provides you with a way of relaxing both mind and body to a remarkable degree. The techniques of inducing self-hypnosis call upon you to focus your attention—to shut out all other distractions, cares, concerns and events in the world around you. The better you are able to do this, the more relaxed and disengaged is your mind. As you will see later, you can use this detached mind in a variety of ways to produce the positive effects you seek. But for the moment, let us remain with the relaxation component.

The pain imprint

Detaching yourself from your pain and things around you, for whatever length of time you wish, enables your mind and body to learn a new set of behaviours. When you have suffered pain for a long while, it can become something of a habit. Your mind develops a pain imprint, something like an integrated circuit in your television set. If your television set breaks down, the technician will often do no more than replace one of the circuits and it will then function perfectly once again. To replace the pain circuit in your brain is not nearly as easy, but developing a regular pattern of physical *and* mental relaxation through self-hypnosis will, in time, help you do this.

One of the main difficulties associated with laboratory investigations of pain relief techniques is that their effectiveness is usually only assessed at the time of the study. Few of them test a patient's response many days later, and yet this is the true measure of the effectiveness of a particular procedure. It is of little benefit if it works when you are doing it but the pain returns to its full intensity the moment you get up and move around. Regular use of self-hypnosis will ensure the continuance of relaxation so that it flows over into each day. Even if you applied self-hypnosis for no other reason than to induce a state of relaxation, that alone would justify its use.

Altering your pain through suggestion

Direct suggestions of pain relief can have a significant effect on how you feel. You are not planning to talk away the pain but simply help your mind *perceive* it in a different way. It will help if you first write down in your work diary (see Chapter 4) the sorts of things you are going to silently communicate to your unconscious. These can be couched in general terms, indicating ways that your body is going to feel and cope in a better manner. Sometimes you may prefer to be more specific and relate them to how a particular area is going to respond. You may, for example, suggest that a joint is going to become less inflamed, cool and more easily moved.

The use of general coping suggestions

As examples of the types of general suggestions you can use, consider the following:

Each day . . . I am going to experience a greater sense of relaxation . . . flowing through each and every part of my body.

As each part relaxes . . . I will notice how much more comfortable . . . and at ease I feel.

And as this general feeling of relaxation . . . starts to build up in my body . . . and become part of me . . . I will notice a much greater sense of comfort . . . coming into my back [or wherever it is you feel most pain].

It will feel so comfortable . . . and so relaxed . . . and those pleasant experiences . . . are going to get stronger . . . and stronger the more I use my therapy.

Gradually . . . I am going to notice . . . the unpleasant feelings flowing away from me . . . and I will find my mind . . . locking in on pleasant thoughts . . . associated with things around me.

I will appreciate each day more . . . enjoying the warmth of the sun . . . the beauty of the flowers in my garden . . . the joy of being with my family and friends.

*I am going to feel so much better about
myself . . . that my interests in my
hobbies . . . family . . . and things around
me will return to the way . . it used to
be.*

*And when I go to bed at night . . . I will
enjoy the feelings of ease . . . warmth . . .
security that I feel as I snuggle down
between the sheets. The feelings of
relaxation . . . and ease that I experience
each day . . . will flow into the night time
. . . so that my sleep is peaceful . . .
restful . . . so enjoyable.*

Constructing specific suggestions

More specific suggestions are phrased in a slightly different
way and you may find it helpful to incorporate them into your
mental imagery. Thus, if you suggest to yourself that a joint
is going to become cooler, less inflamed and less painful, you
can visualise a cool pack around it or imagine it being sprayed
with cool water. The following are guidelines on how you can
construct suggestions appropriatae to your particular pain
problem:

*I feel so relaxed now . . . and in this
relaxed state . . . my mind is so sensitive
to the things that I say.*

*These pleasant feelings of relaxation . . .
are going to flow into the whole of my
body each day . . . and bring with them
so much ease . . . and comfort.*

*The feelings of comfort . . . will feel just
as though they are collecting around my
ankle [you can be specific about the joint
you wish to treat] . . . and they are going
to take over . . . from the unpleasant
sensations.*

*As this happens more and more each day
. . . so my body's defences . . . are going
to get stronger . . . and will fight the
inflammation there.*

*And so my joint is going to feel cooler . . .
and more comfortable. It may be a little
stiff for a while [it is important to be
realistic in your aims] . . . but gradually
. . . that too, will loosen up . . . and feel
so much easier.*

*I can feel my joint becoming cool . . . and
comfortable now . . . as I picture a cold
pack being applied to it. It feels so good
. . . if feels relaxed.*

Using your mental imagery

The second strategy you can use in order to alter your pain experience is to call upon your mental imagery. Unfortunately, not everyone has the same ability to visualise things—either in everyday life or in self-hypnosis—but most of us can see things in our mind's eye to some degree.

Even if your mental imagery is not strong at first, be patient and practise it, for it does get better with reinforcement. Sometimes you may find that your mental pictures cannot be sustained—they seem to come and go. Again, do not be too concerned. Constant practice will train your mind to 'hold' the images for longer and longer periods of time. To get the most out of your self-hypnotic imagery, try as best you can to 'feel' the situation as if it is actually occurring. You can make your mental experiences more vivid by remembering a similar situation from the past, and then imagining it happening to you again. If you adopt the approach of feeling-remembering-thinking and experiencing the particular scene or sensation, you will find that your imagery becomes far more intense, and consequently more beneficial.[54]

There are a great many ways you can use your imagery in self-hypnosis in order to change the way your mind perceives pain. You will find it helpful to explore each one so that you can determine which is going to prove the most useful for *you*. In any case, most patients like to have a number of pain-coping strategies to call upon because it introduces variety and interest into their self-treatment. Monotony can often lead to your becoming less involved in your self-hypnotic techniques.

Changing your mental pain colour

Once you have achieved as deep a level of mental disengagement as possible, a state where you 'let go' of all outside concerns and problems, imagine your pain as a large red disc. Then think of the colour changing gradually to pink and finally, to a complete whiteness. As this change slowly occurs, give yourself the suggestions that your pain is becoming less severe as the red fades to a less intense colour. By the time it has become white you may find that your pain has diminished to a point where it no longer bothers you.

The use of this colour-change technique is well illustrated by Mrs H. She experienced severe pain in her lower back and right groin following a motor accident, in which she fractured several bones in her lower spine. She had a spinal fusion performed to repair this damage and also underwent a hysterectomy several years later. Subsequently she developed adhesions in her abdomen which led to another operation.

There was no apparent cause for her disabling pain and all attempts at relief, including nerve blocks, were of little help. She was aware that the pain had caused her to become tense and stressed. At times, she felt tearful and depressed, had difficulty in sleeping and was concerned because her relationship with her husband had deteriorated. Whereas they used to be very happy together, they now argued a lot and she had lost all interest in love-making.

Apart from being treated in hypnosis, she became a dedicated user of self-hypnosis and found that she was able to control her symptoms very successfully using various pain control strategies. Her favourite one was the colour change technique, and she described her approach in the following way:

> *I see the pain as a red colour and then*
> *gradually change it to pink as the pain*
> *comes down and then to white. At that*
> *stage, I tell the nerves, muscles and blood*
> *vessels to calm down and be normal. After*
> *a while, the pain* does *ease down to a*
> *point where I feel I can cope again.*

Using self-hypnotic techniques on a regular basis has enabled her to lead a perfectly normal life. She is able to run her own business in addition to coping satisfactorily with family commitments, and is rarely troubled now by her pain problem.

Your pain-dimmer switch

In using imagery scenes in self-hypnosis, some people like to draw upon mental pictures of things they have encountered in everyday life, while others prefer to let their mind develop its own fantasy experiences. It doesn't matter which of these you use as long as the images are involving and you have the feeling that you are 'there', experiencing it with a sense of vividness.

An example of how you can employ something that is an everyday part of life is the pain-dimmer switch imagery. Most of us have used a light-dimmer switch at one time or another. If you have, you can use the concept for reducing your pain:

> *I imagine a dimmer switch in my brain*
> *. . . it controls the levels of my pain [this,*
> *incidentally, is in keeping with the gate-*
> *control theory of pain discussed earlier].*
>
> *This switch is similar to the light-dimmer*
> *switch I have at home . . . it turns down*
> *the intensity of light from very bright . . .*
> *to being hardly discernible. In the same*
> *way, my pain-dimmer switch is going to*
> *turn down my pain . . . as I relax . . .*
> *and* think *of my pain becoming hardly*
> *discernible.*

*But before I start using this technique . . .
I am going to think . . . of the level of
pain my mind is experiencing. I can do
this by setting up my own pain meter. I
can see the meter in my mind . . . it
measures my pain level. My mental pain
meter is just like a thermometer . . . I can
measure the pain I feel on a scale of 0 to
100 . . . 0 is no pain and 100 the most
severe I could experience. My pain will be
somewhere on this scale . . . and my mind
has the ability to accurately assess
whereabout it lies . . . on this scale.*

*Now I can picture my own dimmer switch
. . . set at this point. I am turning down
the switch . . . very gradually . . . one
point at a time . . . as I relax. At first
. . . I may only move the intensity . . .
down a slight amount . . . but I am not
discouraged by this. With time and
practice . . . I know I will find it easier
. . . to reduce my pain . . . until I reach
the point . . . where it is scarcely
perceptible.*

Soothing through warmth

Another pain alteration technique is to visualise a scene in which
you induce a sense of warmth. Most people associate a feeling
of warmth with ease and tranquillity. We can all remember
sitting in front of a log fire on a cold night or lying on a quiet
beach on a delightfully warm day, and being at peace with the
world. If such scenes can relax us even when we think about
them in day-to-day life, they will have an even greater effect
when they are linked with the quiet state of self-hypnosis. In
fact, visualising yourself in such a scene can induce many
pleasant sensations in both mind and body, and help break the
cycle of pain $\longrightarrow$ tension and stress $\longrightarrow$ more pain which
has built up over time.

Now that I am in a relaxed state . . . I can take myself off to a quiet scene . . . lying on a lovely beach. The sun is warm . . . I feel a gentle breeze blowing over my body. In the background . . . I hear the sound of the surf . . . as it washes up on the beach . . . and then recedes. I can even smell the salty air . . . hear the sounds of seagulls as they glide over the sea. Whenever I move my hands . . . I feel the sand running between my fingers. [It will help you to get a better sense of involvement in any scene if you picture fine details associated with it, such as the ones mentioned.]

As I lie back on my beach towel . . . my eyes closed . . . my mind at peace . . . I notice how pleasantly warm the sun is on my body. The warmth seems to flow into all parts . . . into my skin . . . muscles . . . joints. It is so soothing . . . so relaxing. I can feel the muscles letting go of tension . . . replacing it with warmth and ease. It seems to pervade every part of me. Nothing matters any more . . . just the feeling of gentle calmness . . . all through me.

And as I feel those pleasant sensations . . . gradually coming into my body . . . they are replacing the unpleasant . . . unwanted experiences with a sense of comfort. [You will find it helpful to repeat these thoughts over and over to yourself so that they have greater effect.]

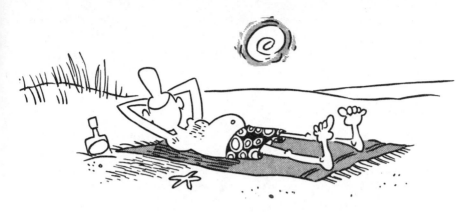

Visualising yourself in a pleasant scene can induce pleasant
sensations

If you do not enjoy lying on a beach there are many other
comforting warm images that you can draw upon. Consider
the following as an example:

*It is a warm . . . peaceful day. I am
lying, face downwards, on a rubber float
. . . in my own pool at home. My eyes are
closed . . . I feel the water flowing gently
between the fingers . . . as I drift slowly
along. How peaceful it all feels . . .
everything in life seems so effortless . . . I
have no cares or worries now . . . only a
feeling of complete ease.*

*The sun feels so pleasantly warm . . . on
my body. I feel it flowing all through me
. . . soothing all the tissues. The tensions
are going . . . being replaced with a sense
of complete ease. Nothing else matters now
. . . only the feelings of total comfort.*

One of the greatest advantages of self-hypnosis is that *you* control how long you spend in it. If you are enjoying the peaceful experiences it brings you, then you can go on using it for as long as you wish. In other words, there are not time constraints in self-hypnosis.

Your pain stop sign

Another technique you can use for altering pain is to visualise a stop sign, similar to ones you see at a road intersection. Some patients find it helpful to use this as a cue mechanism whenever their pain starts to intensify. As with all cue mechanisms, you will need to reinforce it in self-hypnosis by visualising the sign and, at the same time, giving yourself suggestions that whenever you picture it, this will be a signal for the body to relax and feel a sense of ease and warmth. Having a cue mechanism built into your mind, as it were, is not only helpful from a pain-relief standpoint but is also reassuring. There is nothing more frightening and undermining of morale than being constantly afflicted by pain and having no way of dealing with it.

How to distance your mind

While some sufferers like to alter the pain experience, others prefer to use techniques which distract them from it, by involving themselves in other things. There is no limit to the number of these you can use, and you should be guided by the sorts of things you like to do in life. One patient of mine, who was an artist, spent considerable periods of time in self-hypnosis imagining himself painting a scene. He found that this not only helped to develop his painting skills but also reduced his chronic low back pain.

When you use distraction techniques, you usually involve yourself in *active* imagery by picturing yourself *doing* something. Thus, you may recall walking in the countryside, in a forest or along a beach. Alternatively, you may prefer to visualise yourself playing your favourite sport or engaging in a hobby or interest. In order to get the most benefit from this imagery, you should remember what it was like, think about it, and imagine and experience it once again with as much of a sense of involvement as you can muster. As a sample scene, imagine the following:

> *It is early evening . . . I am walking*
> *slowly along a beach. It has been a hot*
> *day . . . but the gentle cooling breeze*
> *blows through my hair . . . bringing me a*
> *sense of relief. I am walking along the*
> *edge of the water . . . I feel it swirling*
> *around my ankles . . . as the tiny waves*
> *wash up on the beach. As each wave goes*
> *out . . . it leaves the sand firm and shiny.*
> *I can even see the sunset reflecting in the*
> *damp sand . . . in pastel shades of blue*
> *and pink.*
>
> *The sun is getting lower now . . . I am*
> *fascinated by the constantly changing*
> *colours of some fluffy clouds on the*
> *horizon. They seem to have a life of their*
> *own . . . one moment white . . . then*
> *changing to a delicate pink . . . and*
> *finally deep magenta.*
>
> *I feel at peace within myself . . . nothing*
> *can bother me in this peaceful scene . . . it*
> *is all so natural . . . so quiet . . . free*
> *from concern.*

Your cocoon of peace

Another procedure which enables you in self-hypnosis to detach yourself from pain for a while is to go into your own inner cocoon of relaxed concentration. This is a variation of Elton's secret room technique[59] and can be especially useful for you if you have difficulty in recalling a scene where you have been pain free. It provides you with a place of security and invulnerability. The value of this cannot be understated if, as many chronic pain sufferers do, you have the feeling that there is nowhere you can go to escape the constant, debilitating feeling. The scene you go into is entirely of your choice.

The cocoon you visualise may be something entirely nebulous, such as swirls of colour. Others like to picture themselves encapsulated in an actual cocoon, like a silkworm. One of my patients, being treated in hospital for severe burns, saw herself ' . . . in a nest, surrounded by my loved ones . . . all of us touching each other'. Whatever your imagery, the aim is to dissociate yourself from the pain experience for a while, to break the constant pain cycle. There could be no more beautiful way to describe the use of this technique than in the words of James Russell Lowell: 'The mind can weave itself warmly in the cocoon of its own thoughts'.

I feel so at ease now . . . completely
relaxed. I am going for a while . . into
my own inner cocoon . . . of relaxed
concentration . . . it is so beautiful there.
In my special cocoon . . . I can experience
. . . whatever pleasant sensations I want
. . . warmth . . . coolness . . . peace.
Nothing can trouble me now . . . I feel
protected . . . insulated . . . from cares
. . . concerns . . . negative thoughts . . .
unwanted feelings. It all feels so good . . .
I am enjoying these moments . . . of
complete ease.

Letting go of your pain

If you have suffered pain for any length of time, you may start to believe that you are *never* going to be free of it. The pain becomes imprinted on your mind and this can have a demoralising effect on you, creating, among other things, a marked loss of self-esteem.

To restate a point I made earlier, it is vital you accept the idea that you *can* influence your pain. Without that belief, in the first instance, it makes it very difficult for you to control your mind, and thus your pain, in a positive way. In other words, you must realise you can let go of your pain rather than having to tolerate it for ever.

One way of achieving this is to literally see yourself letting go of the pain experience. As is the case with all imagery, there are innumerable procedures you can use and these are restricted only by your imaginative capacity. The techniques suggested are only meant as guidelines and you will probably find you adapt them in ways that best suit your particular style and imagery ability.

Your quiet stream

Most of us have, at some time or other, spent a peaceful hour sitting near a stream, enraptured by the sounds it makes as it flows over stones and pebbles. There is an almost hypnotic quality to these sounds of nature and such a scene therefore lends itself beautifully to self-hypnotic imagery. Walker first suggested using the stream imagery as a means of deepening hypnosis,[26] but it can be further expanded so as to allow you to release problems and difficulties.

> *Now that I feel relaxed . . . and*
> *disengaged from the concerns of the world*
> *. . . I am walking along a path . . . that*
> *wends its way through a lovely wood . . .*
> *enjoying the peaceful scene . . . listening*
> *to the birdsong. I am thinking about the*
> *things that bother me . . . about the pain*
> *. . . and how good it would feel to let go of*
> *it. I come to a glade . . . and see a small*
> *stream flowing gently through it. It is so*
> *quiet there . . . and I sit down on the soft*
> *. . . cool . . . grassy bank of the stream*
> *. . . in the shade of a large tree . . .*
> *captivated by the sound of the water . . .*
> *as it trickles and swirls . . . around the*
> *smooth pebbles and stones.*
>
> *I feel at peace . . . in this beautiful scene*
> *. . . there is a gentle breeze rustling the*
> *leaves of the tree . . . some of them drift to*
> *the ground. I pick one up . . . and think*

*of how good it would be . . . if I could put
my pain problem onto that leaf . . . and
let it float right away from me. I will start
. . . by releasing a little bit of the pain
. . . putting it on the leaf . . . placing the
leaf gently on the water . . . and releasing
it. As it floats slowly downstream . . . it is
carrying the pain intensity right away
from my body. It reminds me of a tiny
ship . . . as it bobs this way and that. I
watch . . . the pain getting smaller and
smaller . . . gradually disappearing from
my view . . . I feel more at ease now.*

*Now I can bring my mind back to the
bank of the stream . . . and pick up
another leaf. I would like to release . . .
some other aspect of my pain . . such as
my tiredness. Why not put that on the leaf
. . . and let it float downstream . . . until
it, too, disappears. I can go on . . .
releasing different problems . . . associated
with my pain . . . until it no longer
bothers me.*

Your red balloon

There is something about balloons which appeals to most of
us. Who can fail to remember the pleasure of being given one
as a child. Many an historic event is celebrated with the release
of countless colourful balloons, symbols of joy and freedom.
In view of this, balloon imagery is well suited to use in self-
hypnotic treatment.

*I am now feeling so relaxed . . . so at ease
. . . my mind is no longer troubled by
unwanted thoughts. I can see myself
walking in the countryside . . . I feel at
peace . . . I am strolling through a small
wood . . . and as I emerge from it . . . I*

*see a huge red balloon tethered in a field.
It is larger than any balloon I have ever
seen . . . and suspended beneath it is a
small wicker basket.*

*On the ground nearby . . . I see a small
box . . . it is quite empty. This is a box
into which I can put all the problems . . .
that I would like to release. I can place
my pain . . . into the box . . . and any
other symptoms or difficulties . . . I feel
ready to release. [Only put some pain
into your box. It would be inappropriate
to try to remove it all.]*

*Now that I have placed part of my pain
into the box . . . I am putting it into the
basket. I already feel more at ease . . .
content that I can let go of my pain . . .
and other difficulties.*

*I am setting the balloon free . . .
watching it float higher and higher . . .
into the clear blue sky . . . until it
becomes a tiny red dot . . and then
disappears. My mind and body . . . feel
easier now . . . I have let go of some of my
pain. I am not concerned that I cannot
release it all . . . each time I imagine my
red balloon . . . I will be able to let go of
a little more.*

A delightful variation of this was suggested by a patient and
serves to demonstrate how you can develop your own imagery
techniques. She imagined herself floating upwards in a red hot-
air balloon and, at a certain height, she threw some features
of her pain overboard just as you would release ballast. This
caused her balloon to soar even higher, and gave her the feeling
that she was rising above her pain and freeing herself from
all of its constrictions.

Getting active again

Once your suffering starts to diminish, you will probably experience a desire to return to everyday activities. But what you must realise is that your chronic pain will have caused you to avoid certain patterns of movement, and even simple exercise. Without being aware of it, you will have made certain postural adjustments so as to reduce discomfort and this, in turn, can lead to muscle spasm or a wasting of muscles from disuse.

Before you start mobilising muscles and joints which have been relatively inactive for a long time, it is worth seeking professional advice from a physiotherapist. Failure to do so may result in further damaging your joints or soft tissues, and lead to the undoing of weeks of work on your part. Progress is necessarily slow and so you must be patient, but be encouraged by the fact that any movement you regain will help to restore the normal functioning of the pain-sensing mechanism and prevent the return of the pain.[60]

Up to this point, you have seen how self-hypnosis can help you gain control over the pain factor. It also has a role to play in your rehabilitation, for its continuing use will ensure a greater degree of body relaxation, and aid the return of flexibility in muscles and mobility in joints.

You can use suggestions in self-hypnosis to reinforce your progress in exercise patterns such as walking, swimming or stretching. Imagery rehearsal in self-hypnosis can also be of enormous benefit to you. Spend a little time each day in self-hypnosis, visualising yourself engaging in certain tasks, whether they be household chores, gardening or playing with a child. Remember, a picture is worth a thousand words and your use of such a mental picture will go a long way towards promoting a better sense of wellbeing and a greater ability to be active. One final point needs to be emphasised. It is not sufficient to imagine yourself performing certain activities. They must also be tried out in daily life. It bears repeating that progress will, of necessity, be slow, so be patient. See each small gain in movement as a stepping stone to free activity.

Headaches: their prevention and treatment

There are three reasons why headaches deserve special mention. First, they are a prominent symptom or manifestation of tension and stress; second, they are common, and third, they are amenable to treatment.

It is difficult to assess the prevalence of headache in the general community due to the fact that many headache sufferers do not consult their doctor about them. What we do know is that migraine, for example, has been shown to affect up to 20 per cent of the population.[4]

You will find it easier to learn how to cope with your pain if you understand, in the first instance, what brings it about. There are two broad categories of headache: the tension (or muscular contraction) type and the migrainous variety.

Tension headaches

Tension headaches are, as the term suggests, brought about by stress.[3] This causes a spasm in certain muscle groups in the neck and scalp. Spasm causes pain, and people variously describe the sensation they have as tightness at the back of the head and neck, pressure feelings in the centre of the scalp, a band-like sensation around the whole head or a fullness in the region of the forehead and temple. Quite often, this type of headache will respond to aspirin or paracetamol, but though these drugs will temporarily ease your pain, you would do well to remember that the underlying cause is still there. What your mind is trying to tell you is that it is under pressure and overloaded—in other words, you are stressed.

Migraine

Migraine is often described as a vascular headache. This is because the pain you experience is brought about by certain changes in blood vessels that supply the brain and the head. The first change to occur is a narrowing of these vessels, and this can lead to visual problems, a sensation of numbness in the head or arms and nausea. These symptoms come on before you actually experience the headache. The narrowing or constriction phase is usually short-lived and is followed by a dilatation of these arteries. It is at this stage that the full-blown headache occurs. It can be extremely intense and incapacitating, and often the sufferer has to retire to bed. It tends to be focused over one side of the head and is frequently associated with nausea or vomiting. The severity of the pain is such that people often graphically describe it with phrases like 'I thought my head was going to burst open'.

How stress brings on migraine

Although you may have inherited your predisposition to these attacks, it is also true that stress plays a significant role in their genesis. A typical example of this are the 'weekend migraines' which some experience. Invariably, the preceding week has been stressful. Business pressures and worries may have been excessive and so you go home with the intention of having a relaxing weekend, only to find that you are overtaken by a headache of massive proportions. A question posed by many is 'Well, if stress is the cause of my migraine, why didn't I get it during the week?' The answer lies in your fight-and-flight mechanism. When you are busy, your body is working under an adrenaline effect and so you cope. Once this wears off, the stress persists and you succumb with a headache.

How to manage your headache

Even though stress is a common factor in both tension and migraine headaches, it is important to distinguish what type you experience, for this will determine your best treatment approach. Before you embark on any form of self-therapy, however, consult your physician. While it is likely that your headaches are being caused by muscle contraction, occasionally they signify the presence of something more serious, and this possibility must be eliminated before you set out to treat them. Furthermore, your doctor is in a better position to diagnose the nature of your pain. Armed with this knowledge, you will be in a better position to treat your stress and the effects it is having on you.

The general feelings of relaxation produced through self-hypnosis will have marked beneficial effects on both varieties of headache by reducing your stress. In this sense, it becomes a preventative or prophylactic technique and may be so effective that you have no need to use any other self-hypnotic procedures. If the pain attacks recur then there is an obvious need to employ more specific strategies, depending on your type of headache. In both, the golden rule is to endeavour to use your therapy *as early as possible* in the attack. Once your pain has become established, especially with migraine, it is very difficult to halt its progress.

Treating the tension headache

Frequent tension headaches can be very distressing. They interfere with your enjoyment of life, your powers of concentration and even your sleep. Once you have recognised that they are stress-related, however, you are well on the way to treating them.

Keeping a log in your work diary of their frequency, intensity and the possible stressors that may have precipitated each attack will help you modify certain aspects of your life so that you can control these stressful factors.

Negative self-talk, such as 'Here comes my headache again. I know it is going to be a bad one. I hope I can manage to get through my work,' can also add to stress. These negative thoughts are usually brought on by the start of a headache and serve to further intensify it. This is more likely to happen if you suffer frequent attacks. Be on the look-out for these negative inner conversations and replace them with coping suggestions: 'I can feel the headache coming on. I must be stressed by something. I will sit down for a while and relax using my self-hypnosis. I know that, as I relax, my headache will gradually disappear and I will feel comfortable again.'

You may find your tension headache starts in a situation such as work, where you cannot slip away and do self-hypnosis. This is where the use of a relaxation cue (thinking of the word 'calm' as you breathe out, for example) can be most helpful. If that cue mechanism has been reinforced by constant repetition, it will allow you to call upon it to reduce stress whenever you wish.

The role of mental imagery

Apart from the relaxation aspects of self-hypnosis, you will find specific imagery to be a valuable way of easing the muscle spasm in your head. The most effective imagery is usually associated with inducing a sensation of warmth, the method you employ being determined by what you find works best for you. One of my patients, for example, imagines that he is standing under a hot shower and he maintains this image until the pain is eased. You may wonder why he does not simply stand under a shower, and not bother with self-hypnosis. The answer, of course, lies in the mental relaxation that therapy induces, in addition to the imagery of warmth.

Coping with migraine

If you are a migraine sufferer, the chances are that you are already taking a variety of medications, either to treat or prevent the attacks. In spite of these, your pain may still recur from time to time. Sometimes these bouts are triggered by hormonal changes such as in the premenstrual phase, or by eating the 'wrong' foods, but on occasions they may occur for no apparent reason. If this is happening to you, you can be sure that stress is lurking and needs to be brought under control.

Self-hypnosis will enable you to deal with this mental stress. Together with positive self-statements directed towards easing the pain, it can often be sufficient to abort an attack. If an attack is under way, self-hypnotic imagery will certainly reduce its intensity. Interestingly, most migraine sufferers prefer to visualise coolness rather than warmth as a means of producing ease. If this sensation is combined with hand warming, it produces a marked improvement in pain control. The following imagery and suggestion has been adapted from a technique described by Spiegel and Spiegel (1978), and is one which should offer you a great deal of help in bringing your migraine attacks under control. As has been emphasised so often, feel free to modify it so that it suits your own imaginal capacity.

*Now that I feel so relaxed . . . I can
imagine a gentle . . . cool . . . mist . . . all
around my head. It is so soothing . . . I
can feel that mist . . . all around my head
. . . and face . . . breathing in the cool air
. . . it is cooling the air passages . . .
flowing into the sinuses. As that coolness
. . . flows into my head . . . it is soothing
. . . relaxing the blood vessels . . . they
are slowly . . . shrinking down . . . and
feel so much easier. The numbness . . . is
gently replacing . . . the unwanted pain. I
feel the coolness . . . and ease . . . the
numbness . . . spreading all through my
head . . . soothing away the pain. [Repeat
the sensations as often as necessary until
you experience the coolness.]*

*At the same time . . . I can imagine . . . a
pair of lambswool gloves on my hands.
Inside these gloves are tiny electrical
elements . . . which can heat them.
[Imagine these elements as being similar
to an electric blanket.] As I switch on the
heating elements . . . I feel the warmth
. . . the comfort . . . coming in to my
hands . . . and fingers. The hands are
becoming warmer . . . and warmer. [In
the case of both warmth and coolness,
spend as long as you need thinking about
the sensations, remembering and
imagining each one, until you are able to
fully experience it. Make this an
unhurried process.]*

Using two quite different sensations to control pain may seem
paradoxical. Although various theories have been proposed, no
one knows why hand warming is so effective. It does work
however, providing you spend several minutes each day

practising the technique in self-hypnosis at times when you are headache-free.[5] As with any other skill you wish to perfect in life, the more you practise, the better you become.

If you have difficulty experiencing the hand warmth, your use of the cooling imagery will still produce a significant reduction in pain. It should be emphasised that it is difficult to stop a migraine headache with these techniques once it is fully established. They work best if you apply them as early as possible in an attack. In any case, daily use of these self-hypnotic procedures will ensure that you take control over your attacks and gradually you will notice them diminishing in frequency and severity.

CHAPTER EIGHT

MANAGING OTHER HEALTH PROBLEMS

In Chapter 1, I discussed the influence of the mind on certain diseases. These are sometimes known as psychophysiological disorders because stress can play a significant role in causing or exacerbating them. In view of this, it would be appropriate to consider how you can use self-hypnosis to alleviate them.

COPING WITH ASTHMA

The major feature of this disorder is spasm in the air passages (bronchospasm) which makes exhalation a difficult and distressing experience. A number of factors can cause the spasm: infections, allergies, irritation, medications and stress. Although the control of stress would seem to be the principal reason for using self-hypnosis, it will become clear that a more generalised behavioural approach is also indicated.

Monitoring your lung functioning

Most asthmatics would assume that the intensity of their wheezing should provide a good indication of how their lungs are functioning at that particular moment. Thus, if they are wheezing slightly, it is assumed that their lung function is better than if the wheezing is excessive.

Unfortunately, self-assessment, based on the intensity of your wheezing, is not always an accurate measure of your true lung functioning.[61] For this reason, it is important to use a more accurate, objective, measurement and this can be performed by a peak flow meter. This is a relatively inexpensive device into which you blow. It measures the flow of air through your larger air passages in litres per minute, and a low reading indicates a partial obstruction brought about by bronchospasm and the presence of mucus. It should be emphasised that the use of the peak flow meter is best learned under the guidance of your physician.

At various intervals throughout the day, and especially if wheezing is present, you should record your subjective assessment of the degree of wheeze in your work diary. This can be assessed on a nought to ten scale (where nought is no wheezing and ten the most severe you have ever experienced.) At the same time you should enter in your diary the peak flow reading, how you feel, what you were doing when the wheeze started and the situation in which measurements are made. Any medication (including the use of inhalers) should also be recorded.

Easing your distress

Monitoring your asthma in this way will enable you and your physician to identify situations which are associated with an increase or decrease in peak flow measurements. The other advantage of this procedure is that it allows you to recognise high risk situations and events (for example, dust) so that you can take the necessary steps to avoid them. Most importantly, you will feel that you are able to take responsibility for your own lung functioning, and thus control your disorder instead of having it control you.

Desensitising yourself to stress

Now that you have identified the things that stress you and which lead to spasm in your airways, you can embark on desensitising yourself to these using self-hypnosis. You will find it helpful to draw up a hierarchy of situations in your work diary, starting with the least stressful and ending with the one that causes you most breathing distress.

In self-hypnosis, imagine coping with the least disturbing one in a relaxed way—breathing easily and freely. Once that scene has been mastered, you proceed to the next until finally, you can breathe in a relaxed, normal way in all situations. This desensitisation process should be unhurried and, for it to be effective, must be practiced regularly.

The benefits of relaxation

Spasm of the small muscles surrounding your smaller air passages is brought about by overactivity of your sympathetic nervous system. Sometimes this reaction is triggered by stress; at others, by stimuli such as substances to which you are allergic. The relaxation you experience through self-hypnosis will help to dampen-down the increased sympathetic activity and bring ease to your breathing.

Relaxation effects can be intensified by suggestions given in self-hypnosis:

> *I feel so much calmer . . . feel the*
> *relaxation process easing all my air*
> *passages. The cool . . . fresh air . . . is*
> *flowing so easily . . . into my lungs. I can*
> *breathe effortlessly . . . in . . . and out*
> *. . . in . . . and out. The wheeze is*
> *becoming less . . . the tension . . . the*
> *spasm . . . is flowing out of my lungs . . .*
> *out of my body.*

Practising correct breathing

The daily use of self-hypnosis will also enable you to learn correct breathing techniques. Many people are unaware of the correct way to breathe. Often, they utilise chest breathing, which entails pushing out the rib cage as they inhale and releasing it as they breathe out.

In order to gain a better flow of air into your lungs, it is essential that you learn diaphragmatic breathing. The diaphragm is the muscular partition that separates your chest from the abdomen. Correct breathing involves moving your diaphragm downwards as you breathe in and letting it return to its resting position as you breathe out.

You can practice correct (diaphragmatic) breathing much more effectively when you are relaxed. In self-hypnosis, place your hands on your waist and, as you breathe in, feel the hands being pushed *sideways*. Repetition of this technique will soon ensure that it becomes entirely automatic.

Using your imagery

There are many ways you can employ your imagery ability to ease your wheezing and improve lung functioning. One technique is to visualise your lung being like a collapsed balloon and, as you relax, imagine it gradually reinflating.

Another way of reducing the intensity of an asthmatic attack is to imagine yourself in your inner mental place (see Chapter 4), in which the air is warm and moist. Each time you inhale, feel the warm, moist air flowing into the air passages. This imagery has the dual effect of relaxing airways and loosening mucus which has been produced in response to the asthma attack.

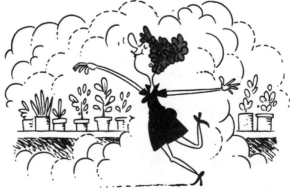

Using imagery during an asthma attack can help improve
lung functioning

THE CONTROL OF HYPERTENSION

A medical check that all of us should undergo each year is the measurement of blood pressure. Why is it desirable to have this regularly assessed? First, prolonged hypertension is one of the major and most correctable of risk factors in coronary heart disease. Second, once it has become established, the internal mechanisms that maintain blood pressure become set at higher and higher levels as time goes by and may prove difficult to reverse.[62]

Altering your behaviour patterns

Having determined that your blood pressure is consistently elevated, your physician will probably prescribe medication which is designed to reduce and maintain it at acceptable levels. In addition to this medication, there is also a great deal *you* can do to control your hypertension.

Controlling your weight is essential (see Chapter 5). If you are overweight, the increased fatty tissue needs to be supplied with a constant blood flow, and the extra demands on the circulation can be sufficient to raise blood pressure. Many studies have shown that losing weight is sufficient, in itself, to control hypertension.[63] Another aspect of diet which you should consider is the reduction of your salt intake. There has been much speculation over the years regarding the importance of this factor, but current opinion indicates that salt restriction is advisable. Caffeine has also been incriminated as a harmful agent and, for this reason, you should restrict your intake of coffee and tea to a minimum.

Alcohol, too, can play a role in elevating your blood pressure, particularly if you drink more than twenty grams of alcohol (two drinks) per day. Studies have demonstrated, for example, a fall in blood pressure when moderately heavy drinkers changed from standard to low alcohol beers.[63]

Finally, the amount of exercise you take must come into consideration. Its importance cannot be overemphasised, for it has been shown that a reduction of blood pressure has occurred after even as little as six weeks of regular training.[64] Admittedly, not everyone is able to embark on something as strenuous as a jogging program, but daily walks of thirty minutes duration lie within the capacity of most of us.

The value of blood pressure monitoring

Taking responsibility for control of your blood pressure is not too difficult once you are aware of the various factors which can elevate it. One of these is stress, and this can play a significant role in the development of hypertension by causing the sympathetic nervous system to constrict blood vessels throughout the body.[65]

Treatment, therefore, should be aimed at reducing the stressful events which cause your blood pressure to rise. But unless you have a means of measuring your blood pressure, self-therapy can often become a matter of guesswork.

Although you may consider the cost of purchasing a sphygmomanometer (the instrument used for measuring blood pressure) to be relatively high, it is outweighed by the health benefits you will experience as a result of its use. Some authorities claim that self-monitoring of your blood pressure can intensify your anxiety about it. Current thinking, however, indicates that it can be beneficial in helping you control your hypertension.[35] It presents one other advantage—that of conditioning you to relax when having your blood pressure recorded. Patients often develop anticipatory stress when measurements are taken by their physician, and this leads to artificially high readings. Frequent self-use of a sphygmomanometer will reduce this concern.[66]

Before you commence using a sphygmomanometer, you should seek guidance from your physician regarding its use and also the ideal levels you should be aiming to achieve. There are no strict guidelines for these, for your 'normal' range will depend upon your age. Blood pressure tends to rise as you get older and what is acceptable at, say, fifty years of age may be considered to be elevated if you were a younger person. As a general rule, however, systolic readings exceeding 140 and diastolic readings in excess of 90 are usually taken to be an indication of hypertension.

It is preferable that you take blood pressure readings at approximately the same time each day and these should be carried out in the seated position, allowing several minutes rest before-hand. Enter the readings in your work diary, together with stressful events which may have contributed to any blood pressure alterations.

Desensitising yourself to stress

Once you have gained an insight into the situations which raise your blood pressure, you are in a better position to desensitise yourself to them using self-hypnotic suggestions and imagery:

> *In this relaxed state . . . my mind . . .*
> *and body feel so calm and at ease. I can*
> *see all things in my life . . . in their*
> *correct perspective now. I am going to be*
> *able to cope . . . much more easily with*
> *[here you suggest the situation or event*
> *which causes you to become stressed] . . .*
> *each day . . . coping with it in a more*
> *relaxed way.*
>
> *As I think about the situation . . .*
> *remember what it was like . . . imagine*
> *myself in it . . . I see myself responding*
> *. . . in a much calmer way . . . feeling*
> *relaxed . . . comfortable. It feels so much*
> *better . . . to respond in this way. I am*
> *smiling . . . my muscles are relaxed . . .*
> *my body loose. I am coping just as I want*
> *to . . . responding in an ideal . . .*
> *satisfactory way. From now onwards . . .*
> *whenever I go into that situation . . . it*
> *will be a signal for me to relax completely*
> *. . . all through my body. [The*
> *suggestions and imagery should be*
> *repeated until you imagine and feel*
> *yourself at ease in that situation.]*

Hand warming imagery

The ultimate aim of self-hypnosis is to help you develop a voluntary control over the blood pressure mechanisms which are normally influenced by your involuntary nervous system. This training effect can only be achieved if you are willing to employ self-hypnotic imagery and suggestions on a daily basis. An approach which will help you reinforce this control is that of hand warming:

> *Now that I feel totally relaxed . . . I*
> *imagine sheepskin-lined gloves . . . snugly*
> *fitting over both my hands. Inside . . .*
> *there are tiny heating elements . . . which*
> *I can control. As I switch on these*
> *elements . . . I feel the warmth . . .*
> *gradually flowing through my hands . . .*
> *my fingers. They feel so comfortable . . .*
> *and relaxed. My blood vessels . . . are*
> *opening up more and more . . . allowing*
> *the blood to flow . . . easily through them.*
> *My blood vessels are dilating . . . in my*
> *hands . . . in my body . . . and my blood*
> *pressure is becoming lower . . . and lower.*
> *[Repeat these suggestions until you*
> *experience warmth in the hands. Visualise*
> *this effect spreading through the body,*
> *dilating all your blood vessels.]*

The use of self-hypnotic techniques, together with changes in other behaviours such as increased exercise, reduction in weight or control of alcohol intake, will ensure you develop an ongoing control over your blood pressure. In some cases, this will result in your being able to cease medication. In others, there may be a need for continuing antihypertensive treatment, but in a reduced dosage. Irrespective of which group you fall in, your gains will have been noteworthy and beneficial to your body.

TREATING SKIN DISORDERS

Many skin conditions are known to be related to stress. They include atopic eczema, neurodermatitis, acne rosacea, psoriasis, alopecia (both partial and total), herpes simplex, warts and pruritis or itching. Stress is the common exacerbating factor in all of these conditions and it follows that the alleviation of this should be the first consideration if you are to rid yourself of any of these skin problems.

Do things get under your skin?

There are many metaphors that we use in our daily speech which have surprising accuracy. How often have you commented upon something or someone 'getting under your skin,' meaning that they irritate you in some way? You may find that you react to this by your skin becoming irritated and you scratch at it or develop a rash or weals in some part of the body.

If you suffer from a chronic skin problem it is very necessary for you to try and identify the things in your life that act as stressors, and then set out to deal with these in an effective way. Whenever your skin problem flares up, you should write down in your work diary the possible things that could have contributed to stress. The list may be extensive but it does, at least, provide a platform for gaining insight into stressors in your life. Once you recognise the things that bother you, you are well on the way towards dealing with them.

The state of self-hypnosis provides you with an ideal medium in which you can look at and work through the problem issues you have written in your work diary. You are in a perfectly relaxed state of mind and body, free from confusing, anxious thoughts. This anxiety-free state allows you the opportunity to view each potential stressor in perspective, and often this will enable you to resolve the particular things that bother you.

The benefits of imagery

In addition to using self-hypnosis to help you gain insight into the stressors in your life, you can employ imagery techniques which will enhance your unconscious control over the skin lesions. As an instance I recall Mrs A., who was a sensitive, intelligent perfectionist. She led a busy life, for in addition to running her own boutique, she was raising a family of four children. Consequently, for years she had been under a great deal of mental pressure. She presented with a total loss of head and body hair (alopecia), which had occurred twice before during the past fifteen years. Her hair had regrown slowly on each occasion in the past but, whenever she experienced significant stress in her life, this led to further hair loss. Her present bout of alopecia, which had been present for three years, had proved resistant to a variety of dermatological approaches.

She proved to have a good insight into the things which troubled her and realised that stress was contributing to her condition. Nevertheless, in spite of these things, she had difficulty in relaxing and coping with her various commitments.

Over a period of nine months, she diligently used the self-hypnotic techniques taught to her. Her mental imagery involved visualising an increased blood supply being carried to all her hair follicles until she was able to feel warmth and tingling in her scalp At the same time, she gave herself suggestions that the increased blood supply would nourish the dormant hair and cause it to grow and become stronger.

Gradually the hair grew, starting as a fine down and then becoming stronger and thicker. Her continuing use of self-hypnosis has reassured her that *she* is now in control of her life rather than her life controlling her. She feels justifiably confident that she will not lose her hair in the future because of her ability to relax and cope more satisfactorily with her life pressures.

Soothing your itch

A common accompaniment of stress-induced skin lesions is itching (pruritus). This can become a chronic problem and the scratching associated with it further damages the skin, often leading to infection. Once the cycle of stress ⟶ pruritus ⟶ scratching has become established, it can prove difficult to resolve.

Appropriate suggestions given in self-hypnosis, together with the use of imagery, can be an effective way of breaking this cycle:

*I feel so relaxed . . . my mind is at ease
. . . my skin feels calm . . . and cool
. . .so calm . . . so cool. I picture myself
lying on a bed . . . of soft . . . cool moss
. . . near a waterfall. A fine spray . . . is
drifting over my body . . . over my [here
you insert the part of the body affected by
the rash]. It is soothing . . . so soothing.
Nothing matters but the feeling of coolness
. . . that I feel. [These suggestions should
be repeated as often as necessary until you
experience an alleviation of the itching.]*

The type of mental imagery you use is determined by your imaginal capacity and you should select the one which engenders the most vivid sensations of ease for you. You may prefer, for example, to imagine floating in a pool of cool water, or being sprayed with a fine cool, oily mist which anaesthetises your irritated skin.

When using these techniques, it is essential that you have realistic expectations concerning your rate of improvement (see Chapter 1). The skin is a complex organ composed of many layers of cells and inevitably, disease will result in changes in all or most of these. It will require time, repetition of relieving techniques and patience before the damaged cells are replaced by healthy ones.

REINFORCING YOUR BODY'S IMMUNITY

Over the past decade, many research studies have demonstrated that stress can reduce your body's immunity system.[8,67] In view of these findings, it would probably not surprise you to learn that relaxation techniques such as self-hypnosis have been shown to increase your defence mechanisms.[68] Since none of us enjoy the prospect of suffering from constant respiratory infections or allergies, and especially of being confronted by cancer, it makes good sense to do everything in our power to reduce stress to a minimum.

But what if you are already a chronic sufferer from respiratory infections, allergies, or have had treatment for cancer? Is there any place for self-hypnosis at this stage? There most certainly is, for by raising the body's defences (see Chapter 1), it can help to treat the disorder which is affecting you.

The self-management of cancer

Because of its serious nature and the degree of emotional distress experienced by sufferers, we can use cancer as a valuable model in order to illustrate the ways in which self-hypnosis can be applied. One of the major benefits of using this technique is that of reducing stress in a cancer patient's life. This leads to a better quality of life and sometimes prolongs survival.[69]

Self-hypnosis enables people who suffer from cancer to experience a greater sense of wellness, optimism and an overall improvement in morale. If it achieved no more beneficial effects than these, its use would be well justified. Quite often, patients describe becoming isolated within their own fears and concerns on learning that they have cancer. They find that they are unable to talk about the disease and its treatment and this leads to them becoming depressed and anxious. Once this state of emotional stress becomes established it only serves to further intensify the progress of the cancer, as well as destroying the will to fight the disease. Self-hypnosis can help cancer patients to break this chain of events so that they can better cope with the illness.

Coping with the side effects of therapy

Treatment of cancer may involve radiotherapy, chemotherapy and/or surgery, the particular therapy selected by your physician being determined by the nature, situation and severity of the cancer. Unfortunately, as valuable and necessary as chemotherapy and radiotherapy are, they do have certain side effects which can be disturbing and stressful. Common distressing side effects are nausea, vomiting, loss of hair, fatigue and loss of appetite. These may be so severe that they cause you to become fearful of attending for further treatment.

If these side effects have been troublesome for you, you will find that the use of self-suggestions and imagery in self-hypnosis can help to minimise them. A case in point was Mr J. who had undergone chemotherapy for the treatment of a lung cancer. Therapy caused him to experience severe nausea and vomiting and he became extremely depressed by his subsequent loss of hair. For all these reasons, he expressed great reluctance to return to hospital for a second course of the drugs. He was taught self-hypnosis and applied these techniques daily, using positive self-statements that he would relax and feel a sense of control over his symptoms. In addition, he employed imagery to increase his coping skills—visualising himself in hospital feeling entirely at ease as he underwent intravenous infusion of the drugs.

If he became aware of being tense, anxious or had a flare-up of his symptoms, he would immediately use a cue mechanism in order to relax, by visualising himself in a very peaceful scene. These self-hypnotic techniques enabled him to attend for further chemotherapy and, in addition, cope far more satisfactorily with its side effects upon returning home.

The value of mental imagery

Another approach to stimulating the immune functioning in the body is through the use of specific imagery in self-hypnosis. Imagery alone can be a most valuable therapeutic tool, but when combined with hypnosis or self-hypnosis it attains a much greater degree of vividness and involvement ('as if you are really there, experiencing it' as one patient so aptly described it).

Some of the early studies on treating cancer with imagery were carried out by the Simontons,[70] and many of their techniques lend themselves for use in self-hypnosis. Having achieved a state of relaxation and quietness of the mind, you can enhance your body's immune processes through the use of the following imagery:

1. Picture your natural-killer cells as being strong and powerful, moving through the blood stream in an army—constantly hunting for cancer cells. Some people like to view these as knights on white chargers or as heavily armed Samurai.
2. Imagine the cancer cells as weak, soft and easily killed.

3. Visualise the short but successful battle that ensues when your natural-killer cells make contact with the enemy.
4. See the broken-down, dead cancer cells being flushed out of the body. (One of my patients visualises the dead cells being put down a chute which carries them to a beach. As the tide comes in it washes them away, leaving the sand white and clean.)
5. Imagine yourself as being healthy, free from cancer and leading a fulfilling life, playing with your children or working around the garden.

In self-hypnosis, you will often find that you spontaneously develop vivid and imaginative techniques to combat the cancer cells. Allowing your mind 'free-play' in this way may prove far more rewarding than trying to guide it into using preselected imagery.

HELPING THE STRESSED CHILD

Although we are usually able to identify stress quite easily in ourselves, it sometimes proves much harder to do so in children. They may present with disorders or problems, such as asthma or behavioural difficulties, which appear to be unrelated to stress. If stress goes unrecognised as being the causative factor, then there is little likelihood of achieving a satisfactory treatment outcome.

Even if children are able to recognise that they are stresed, they may not have the verbal skills or emotional maturity to express how they feel. Nature has compensated for this by enabling them to express their distress in a more tangible way— through a symptom, a disorder or by producing changes in behaviours. The latter may include such things as disobedience, a drop in academic standards or disruptive behaviours in class. Often, the stress leads to their flouting authority, especially that of parents, and the resultant clashes further fuel the problem.

The problems of parenting

Every child has a deep and constant need for security, and the most important 'anchors' in a child's life are the parents. It is not surprising, therefore, that stress in a parent or dissension at home between mother and father can readily cause the child to become insecure and stressed.

The role of parents in preventing their child becoming stressed is one that cannot be overemphasised. Good parenting is certainly not an easy task and it is one that, in spite of its importance, is invariably learnt through trial and error. There are no training courses which teach us how to parent, nor are there examinations which assess our suitability. Perhaps if there were, most of us would fail.

Listening to your child

The essence of good parenting is to be 'tuned in' to your child. When children wish to discuss something which is bothering them, it is usually introduced in a casual manner and is often concealed in general issues which bear no relevance to the real issue. A child is unlikely to state, for example, 'You know Mum, the thing that bothers me most is that other children make fun of me at school'. But if you realise your child is trying to tell you something, gentle probing questions will usually uncover what it is that is troubling him or her.

The most important thing for you to realise is that *your child* selects the appropriate moment to tell you about the problem. It may have taken considerable time for the young person to muster enough courage to voice concern. If you postpone that opportunity to talk with your child by saying such things as 'I am busy now; talk to me after I have prepared dinner', the child will interpret this as lack of interest on your part. You will have missed a wonderful opportunity to help reduce your child's stress. So the golden rule for listening to children must be: the moment is *now*.

The broken home

If a secure family constellation is so necessary for a child, should parents try to maintain a pretence of happiness even though they are in a position of unresolvable conflict? It is not possible to give an authoritative answer to this question because, obviously, each situation must be considered on its merits.

Probably the most essential things for estranged parents to ensure is that the love they feel for their child is clearly demonstrated by both, is unconditional, and the child is not called upon to act as an adjudicator between them. Most children prefer to take a neutral position when parents are in dispute, and asking them to do otherwise can be confusing and stressful for them.

Jane was a perfect example of how domestic disharmony can create a stress-related disorder in a child. She was an intelligent, artistic twelve-year-old who, for the past two years, had suffered from bouts of bleeding from her bowel. Complex investigations had revealed no obvious physical cause to account for her continuing problem.

Her illness caused her to miss a great deal of schooling and her examination results were therefore poor. She harboured many concerns about her future security. Her parents had been in conflict for many years and were openly discussing the possibility of divorce. She felt great love for them both but her father was so preoccupied with his own concerns that he failed to demonstrate sufficient love and understanding for her. She felt rejected by him and was distressed by what was happening to her formerly secure home environment.

Even though her parents subsequently divorced, relaxation through hypnotic and self-hypnotic therapy enabled her to gain a better perspective on home problems. She was able to confront the situation more easily and understand why her parents had had to pursue their particular course of action. This resulted in a resolution of her bleeding and a return to good health.

School phobia

A child's stress arising from parental disharmony, or from one of the parents being stressed, sometimes results in the child developing a school phobia. This term would suggest that a child is fearful of going to school. In a small percentage of children suffering from this condition this may, indeed, be the case. It can stem, for example, from conflict with a teacher or being bullied by peers. In most cases of school phobia, however, the *real* reason is that the child is more fearful of leaving home (because of insecurities there), rather than of going to school.

The child may be concerned about leaving mother on her own, fearful that she will not be able to cope. This can be the source of intense stress in the young person and a variety of strategies will be employed by the child to ensure that mother is not left unsupported. Treatment of this problem, as with so many others related to children, involves a two-pronged approach—dealing with stress both in the parents and in the child.

Self-hypnosis and children

Children possess two important characteristics which make them excellent subjects for hypnosis. The first is their ability to fantasise and 'lose' themselves in an imagined scene. Secondly, they enjoy experiencing new adventures, provided, of course, that they are safe and non-threatening.

If children are such good subjects in hypnosis, it would be reasonable to assume that self-hypnosis should also be of considerable value. Unfortunately, this is not always the case, for a child who is stressed is often reluctant to practise it, tending to view it as just one more form of discipline and regimentation. If a child is actively resistant to its use it is best to respect his or her wishes. Most children are receptive, however, to the idea of using simple relaxation techniques, or a relaxation cue mechanism (see Chapter 4) which they can apply whenever they feel distressed.

Helping the younger child

The techniques employed by children in learning to relax will depend upon their age. Younger children (below the age of ten years) are best taught relaxation through the use of imaginal techniques. At first, it will be necessary for them to be helped by a parent and, because young people have a shorter attentional span than adults, the relaxation session should not exceed ten minutes.

John was a seven-year-old whose parents were divorced. His principal problem was soiling, which started about a year after the breakdown of his parents' marriage. His mother was a sensitive and perceptive person but, as is common in single parents, endeavoured to compensate for the lack of a father figure by giving him excessive attention.

She had sought medical advice about his disorder but no bowel abnormality was detected. Clearly, she was extremely distressed by its persistence and this only served to intensify the child's problem. Therapy was directed at two levels: to help his mother realise the importance of developing a more relaxed attitude to her child and his disorder, and to reducing her son's concerns.

The first step was to teach his mother how to induce relaxation in her child. Each day, she set aside ten minutes for the relaxation exercises. These were carried out with her sitting on a carpetted floor and John lying beside her. He was asked to close his eyes as if going to sleep and then told to think about lots of different coloured balloons floating in the air, attached to each other by long pieces of string. When he was able to picture these, he nodded his head.

Next, his mother suggested he could release one of the balloons (for example, a red one) by untying the string and watch it float high into the sky. As he watched the balloon float slowly upwards, suggestions were made that he would feel floppy and comfortable all over his body. This procedure was repeated for several minutes with different coloured balloons until John was settled and peaceful.

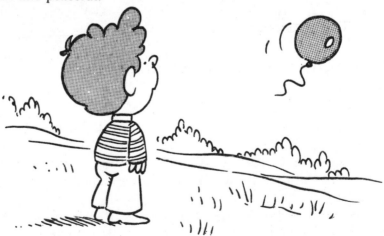

Children can learn relaxation through imagined techniques such as floating balloons

Finally, his mother gave him suggestions that, if he wished, he could attach to the end of a string something that was worrying him, and watch that float away too.

This simple, yet effective, imaginal procedure enabled mother and son to spend quiet moments together, helped John to relax and demonstrated to him that he need no longer be troubled by his concerns. The symptoms gradually subsided and, after several months, had resolved.

Helping the older child

Whereas young children need the involvement of a parent, older ones usually prefer to use self-hypnotic techniques on their own. But a child, whatever the age, is unlikely to spend time applying these techniques unless first, he or she understands the reasons for doing so. The concept of worry is not an easy one for a child to grasp. The role of the parents is to talk to the young person about how pleasant it is to relax. Emphasise the beneficial effects, such as being able to concentrate better on schoolwork and sport, feeling less upset when things go wrong and having more energy. Select problems which you have identified in your offspring and suggest that they will cope with these far more easily if relaxed.

Some teenage children are able to employ adult techniques as means of inducing relaxation. Others are more comfortable in using modifications of these procedures. The techniques they choose should be simple, easily remembered and, preferably, involve active imagery. One that most children find helpful and absorbing is the use of floating leaves.[26]

> As I rest . . . and close my eyes . . . I
> picture myself resting quietly . . . on the
> soft, grassy bank of a little stream. I am
> sitting in the shade of a large tree. It is a
> warm day . . . and it feels nice . . .
> listening to the sounds of the water . . . as
> it trickles over the smooth pebbles and
> stones.

There is a gentle breeze blowing . . .
rustling the leaves of the trees. Some of the
leaves . . . are drifting down to the
ground. I pick up one of the leaves . . .
and drop it onto the water . . . watch it
float slowly downstream. As it floats
further . . . and further away from me
. . . I feel so much more relaxed. It is
getting smaller . . . and smaller . . . and I
am becoming more . . . and more relaxed.

Now it has disappeared from my view
. . . and I pick up another leaf . . . drop
it into the stream . . . and watch it . . .
gently float away from me. Everything
feels so peaceful . . . so quiet. (The child
can continue to drop leaves into the
stream until completely relaxed.)

Once the child feels relaxed, this technique can be further utilised to release concerns and worries. The parents should explain that it is not necessary to cling on to problems. It is far more sensible to let go of these, and this can be achieved by placing each one on a leaf and letting it float away. Children have such excellent imaginal powers that they are able to use this technique to great effect.

CONCLUDING THOUGHTS

Through this book I have endeavoured to acquaint you with ways in which stress can undermine the health of your body and mind. But gaining an understanding of these harmful effects is of little value unless you develop means of treating and, more importantly, preventing them.

For most people, stress arises from everyday hassles rather than from larger events. Self-hypnosis enables you to utilise your own natural talents so that you can cope more effectively with these events in your life. Once you have learnt self-hypnotic skills, they will put few demands on your time and the effort you put into them will surely be rewarded by better health and a continuing sense of peace.

REFERENCES

1 'Exercise and Endorphin' *British Medical Journal*, 30 June 1984, 1950.
2 Webster I. W. 'The Stress Industry', *Australian Doctor Weekly*, 11 Sept. 1987.
3 Jackson, J. A. 'Tension Headaches: Options for treating stress and anxiety', *Patient Management*, Aug. 1984, 63–69.
4 Selby, G. *Migraine and its variants*. Sydney: Adis Health Science Press, 1983.
5 Brown, D. P. & Fromm, E. *Hypnosis and Behavioral Medicine*, 102. New Jersey: Lawrence Erlbaum Associates, 1987.
6 Purcell, K. & Weiss, J. H. 'Asthma', In C. G. Costello (Ed.), *Symptoms of psychopathology*, 597–623, New York. Wiley, 1970.
7 Kirsner, J. B. & Palmer, W. L. 'The irritable colon'. *Gastroenterology*, 1985, *34*, 491–501.
8 Riley, V. M., Fitzmaurice, M. A. & Spackman, D. H. 'Psychoneuro-immunologic factors in neoplasia: studies in animals'. In Robert Ader (Ed.) *Psychoneuroimmunology*, 31–102. New York. Academic Press, 1981.
9 Fromm, E., Leichtman, J. & Brown, D. 'Similarities and differences between heterohypnosis and self-hypnosis: A phenomenological study'. Paper presented at the 25th annual meeting of the Society for Clinical and Experimental Hypnosis, 1973.
10 Fromm, E., Brown, D. P., Hunt, S. W., Oberlander, J. Z. Boxer, A. M. & Pfeifer, G. The phenomena and charactersitics of self-hypnosis. *International Journal of Clinical and Experimental Hypnosis*, 1981, *29*, 189–246.
11 Clark, J. C. & Jackson, J. A. *Hypnosis and behavior therapy: The treatment of anxiety and phobias*. New York: Springer Publishing Co, 1983.
12 Hilgard, J. R. *Personality and Hypnosis: A study of imaginative involvement*. Chicago: University of Chicago Press, 1970.
13 Rawlings, R. M. *The genetics of hypnotisability*. Unpublished honours thesis. University of N.S.W. January, 1977.
14 Spiegel, H. & Spiegel, D. *Trance and treatment: Clinical uses of hypnosis*. New York: Basic Books, 1978.
15 Mitchell, G. P. & Lundy, R. M. 'The effects of relaxation and imagery inductions on responses to suggestions'. *International Journal of Clinical and Experimental Hypnosis*, 1986, *34*, 98–100.
16 Jencks, B. 'Utilizing the phases of the breathing rhythm in hypnosis'. In F. H. Frankel & H. S. Zamansky (Eds)., *Hypnosis at its bicentennial*, 169–181, New York: Plenum Press, 1978.
17 Benson, H. *The relaxation response*. New York: William Morrow, 1975.
18 Stanton, H. E. 'Patient-controlled hypnotherapy: One answer to resistance?' *Australian Journal of Clinical and Experimental Hypnosis*, 1980, *8*, 91–94.
19 Ellis, A. & Harper, R. A. *A new guide to rational living*. Englewood Cliffs, N.J.: Prentice Hall, 1975.
20 Meichenbaum, D. *Cognitive behavior modification: an integrative approach*. New York: Plenum Press, 1977.
21 Salter, A. 'Three techniques of autohypnosis'. *Journal of General Psychology*, 1941, 24, 423–438.

22   Hartland, J. *Medical and dental hypnosis and its clinical applications.* London: Balliere Tindale, 1971.
23   Elton, D., Stanley, G. & Burrows, G. *Psychological control of pain,* p. 135–137. Sydney: Grune & Stratton, 1983.
24   Walker, W. L. The secret room for problem solving. *Australian Journal of Clinical and Experimental Hypnosis,* 1981, *9,* 102–103.
25   Stanton, H. E. 'Elaborations on Elton's "secret room".' *Australian Journal of Clinical and Experimental Hypnosis,* 1979, *7,* 283–285.
26   Walker, W. L. 'Going further with floating leaves—an imagery-based deepening teachnique'. *Australian Journal of Clinical and Experimental Hypnosis,* 1982, *10,* 74–75.
27   Levis, D. J. & Hare, D. J. 'A review of the theoretical rationale and empirical support for the extinction approach of implosive (flooding) therapy.' In M. Hersen, R. M. Eisler & P. M. Miller (Eds), *Progress in behavior modification,* New York: Academic Press, 1977.
28   Kornauser, A. *The mental health of the industrial worker,* New York. Wiley, 1965.
29   Cobb, S. & Rose, R. M. Hypertension, peptic ulcer and diabetes in traffic controllers. *Journal of the American Medical Association,* 1973, *224,* 489–492.
30   Friedman, M., & Rosenman, R. H. *Type A behavior and your heart.* New York: Knopf, 1974.
31   'Coronary-prone behavior and coronary heart disease: A critical review.' *Circulation,* 1981, *63,* 1199–1215.
32   Case, R. B., Heller, S. S., Case, N. B. & Moss, A. J. 'Type A behavior and survival after acute myocardial infarction'. *The New England Journal of Medicine,* 1985, *312,* 737–741.
33   Bauer, G. E. 'Screening and diagnostic evaluation of the hypertensive patient'. *Patient Management,* 1978, *2,* 8–9.
34   Whitehead, W. E., Blackwell, B., DeSilva, H. & Robinson, A. 'Anxiety and anger in hypertension'. *Journal of Psychosomatic Research,* 1977, *21,* 383–389.
35   Jackson, J. A. 'Hypnosis in the treatment of a hypertensive patient: A longitudinal study'. *Australian Journal of Clinical and Experimental Hypnosis,* 1979, *7,* 199–206.
36   Backus, F. I. & Dudley, D. L. 'Observations of psycho-social factors and their relationship to organise disease'. In D. R. Lipsitt & P. C. Whybron (Eds), *Psychosomatic Medicine,* 187–203. New York: Oxford Univ. Press, 1977.
37   Cooper, K. H. *The new aerobics.* New York: Bantam Books, 1972.
38   Fox, S. J. 'Relationship of activity habits to coronary heart disease'. In J. Naughton & H. K. Hellerstein (Eds), *Exercise testing and exercise training in coronary heart disease.* New York: Academic Press, 1973.
39   Brischetto, C. S., Connor, W. E. & Connor, S. L. 'Plasma lipid and lipoprotein profiles of cigarette smokers from randomly selected families'. *American Journal of Cardiology,* 1983, *52,* 675–680.
40   Rosenberg, L., Kaufman, D. W. & Helmaich, S. P. 'The risk of myocardial infarction after quitting smoking in men under 55 years of age'. *New England Journal of Medicine,* 1985, *313,* 1511–1514.
41   Abbott, R. D., Yin, Y. & Reed, D. M. 'Risk of stroke in male cigarette smokers'. *New England Journal of Medicine,* 1986, *315,* 717–720.

42 Fixx, J. F. *The complete book of running.* p. 10. Collingwood, Vic: Outback Press Pty Ltd, 1978.

43 Collins, J. K., Jupp, J. J. & Krass, J. 'Hypnosis and weight control: A preliminary report in the Macquarie University programme'. *Australian Journal of Clinical and Experimental Hypnosis*, 1981, *9*, 93–99.

44 Bauer, G. E. 'Alcohol consumption and arterial hypertension: Epidemiology, mechanisms and management'. In M. L. Wahlqvist & A. S. Truswell (Eds), *Recent advances in clinical nutrition.* London: John Libbey, 1986.

45 Evans, F. J. 'Sleep, eating, and weight disorders'. In R. K. Goodstein (Ed.), *Eating and weight disorders.* New York: Springer Publishing Co., 1983.

46 Holmes, T. H. & Rahe, R. H. The social readjustment rating scale. *Journal of Psychosomatic Research*, 1967, *11*, 213.

47 Carruthers, M. & Taggart, P. Paleocardiology and neocardiology. *American Heart Journal*, 1974, *88*, 1–6.

48 Naruse, G. The hypnotic treatment of stage fright in champion athletes. *International Journal of Clinical and Experimental Hypnosis*, 1965, *3*, 63–70.

49 Patmore, A. *Playing on their nerves: The sport experiment.* London: Stanley Paul & Co. Ltd, 1979.

50 *Greg Norman's golf clinic.* A teaching videotape recording. Austsport production.

51 Suinn, R. M. 'Relaxation control and peak performance'. Paper read at the Association for the Advancement of Behavior Therapy, 1980.

52 Nideffer, R. M. 'The relationship of attention and anxiety to performance'. In W. F. Straub (Ed.), Sport psychology: *An analysis of athlete behavior.* New York: Mouvement Publication, 1978.

53 Unestahl, L. E. *Hypnotic preparation of athletes.* The Department of Sport Psychology. Orebro University, Sweden, 1979.

54 Barber, T. X. 'Changing "unchangeable" bodily processes by (hypnotic) suggestions: A new look at hypnosis, cognitions, imagining, and the mind-body problem.' In A. A. Sheikh (Ed.), *Imagination and Healing.* New York: Baywood Publishing Co. Inc., 1984.

55 Health survey conducted by the Australian Bureau of Statistics, 1977–88. In *The impact of arthritis on the Australian community.* A paper prepared for Charles E. Frosst (Australia) Pty Ltd 1982.

56 Melzack, R. & Wall, R. D. Gate control theory of pain. In A. Soulairac, J. Cahn & J. Charpentier (Eds), *Pain.* London: Academic Press, 1968, 11–200.

57 Shor, R. E. 'Physiological effects of painful stimulation during hypnotic analgesia under conditions designed to minimize anxiety'. *International Journal of Clinical and Experimental Hypnosis*, 1962, *10*, 182–202.

58 Elton, D. & Stanley, G. V. Relaxation as a method of pain control. *Australian Journal of Physiotherapy*, 1976, *221*, 121–123.

59 Elton, D, Stanley G. & Burrows, G. *Psychological control of pain.* Sydney: Grune & Stratton, 1983, 135–137.

60 Melzack, R. *The puzzle of pain.* New York: Basic Books, 1973.

61 Chai, Hyman, Purcell, Kenneth, Brady, Kirk & Falliers. 'Therapeutic and investigational evaluation of asthmatic children'. *Journal of Allergy*, 1968, *41*, 23–36.

62 Surwitt, R. S., Williams, R. B. & Shapiro, D. *Behavioral approaches to cardiovascular disease.* New York: Academic Press, 1982.

63 Jennings, G. Non-drug treatment of hypertension. *Australian Prescriber*, 1986, *10*.

64 Horvath, J. S. & Gillin, A. F. 'Should we prescribe exercise for hypertension?' *Patient Management*, May 1987, 183–191.

65 Whitehead, W. E., Blackwell, B., DeSilva, H. & Robinson, A. 'Anxiety anger in hypertension'. *Journal of Psychosomatic Researach*, 1977, *21*, 383–389.

66 Brener, J. & Kleinman, R. A. 'Learned control of decreases in systolic blood pressure'. *Nature*. 1970, *226*, 1063–1064.

67 Sklár, L. S. & Anisman, H. 'Stress and cancer'. *Psychological Bulletin*, 1981, 89, 369–406.

68 Hall, H. R., Longo, S. & Dixon, R. H. 'Hypnosis and the immune system: The effect of hypnosis on T and B cell function'. In A. A. Sheikh (Ed.), *Imagination and healing*, 159–169. New York: Baywood Publishing Co., 1984.

69 Le Baw, W., Holton, C., Tewell, K. & Eccles, D. 'The use of self-hypnosis by children with cancer'. *American Journal of Clinical Hypnosis, 1975, 17*, 233–238.

70 Simonton, O. C., Mathews-Simonton, S. & Creighton, J. L. *Getting well again: A step-by-step, self-help guide to overcoming cancer for patients and their families.* New York: Bantam Books, 1978.

INDEX

NOTES

NOTES

Piatkus Books

If you are interested in health, recovery and personal growth, you may like to read other titles published by Piatkus.

Recovery

Adult Children of Divorce: How to achieve happier relationships
Dr Edward W. Beal and Gloria Hochman (Foreword by Zelda West-Meads of *RELATE*)

At My Father's Wedding: Reclaiming our true masculinity John Lee

Children of Alcoholics: How a parent's drinking can affect your life
David Stafford

The Chosen Child Syndrome: What to do when a parent's love rules your life Dr Patricia Love and Jo Robinson

Codependent's Guide to the Twelve Steps: How to understand and follow a recovery programme Melody Beattie

Codependency: How to break free and live your own life David Stafford and Liz Hodgkinson

Creating Love: The next great stage of growth John Bradshaw

Don't Call it Love: Recovery from sexual addiction Dr Patrick Carnes

Homecoming: Reclaiming and championing your inner child John Bradshaw

Obsessive Love: How to free your emotions and live again Liz Hodgkinson

When Food is Love: Exploring the relationship between eating and intimacy Geneen Roth

Health

Acupressure: How to cure ailments the natural way Michael Reed Gach

The Alexander Technique: How it can help you Liz Hodgkinson

Aromatherapy: The encyclopedia of plants and oils and how they help you Danièle Ryman

Arthritis Relief at Your Fingertips: How to use acupressure massage to ease your aches and pains Michael Reed Gach

The Encyclopedia of Alternative Health Care: The complete guide to choices in healing Kristin Olsen

Healing Breakthroughs: How your attitudes and beliefs can affect your health Dr Larry Dossey

Herbal Remedies: The complete guide to natural healing Jill Nice

Hypnosis Regression Therapy: How reliving early experiences can improve your life Ursula Markham

Increase Your Energy: Regain your zest for life the natural way Louis Proto

Infertility: Modern treatments and the issues they raise Maggie Jones

Nervous Breakdown: What is it? What causes it? Who will help? Jenny Cozens

Psycho-Regression: A new system for healing and personal growth
Dr Francesca Rossetti
The Reflexology Handbook: A complete guide   Laura Norman and Thomas
Cowan
Self-Healing: How to use your mind to heal your body   Louis Proto
The Shiatsu Workbook: A beginners' guide   Nigel Dawes
Spiritual Healing: All you need to know   Liz Hodgkinson
Super Health: How to control your body's natural defences   Christian
H. Godefroy
Super Massage: Simple techniques for instant relaxation   Gordon Inkeles
The Three Minute Meditator   David Harp
Women's Cancers: The treatment options   Donna Dawson

Personal Growth

**Be Your Own Best Friend: How to achieve greater self-esteem and
happiness**   Louis Proto
**Care of the Soul: How to add depth and meaning to your everyday
life**   Thomas Moore
Colour Your Life: Discover your true personality through colour
Howard and Dorothy Sun
**Creating Abundance: How to bring wealth and fulfilment into your
life**   Andrew Ferguson
**Dare to Connect: How to create confidence, trust and loving
relationships**   Susan Jeffers
Fire in the Belly: On being a man   Sam Keen
Living Magically: A new vision of reality   Gill Edwards
**The Passion Paradox: What to do when one person loves more than
the other**   Dr Dean C. Delis with Cassandra Phillips
**Protect Yourself: How to be safe on the streets, in the home, at work,
when travelling**   Jessica Davies
The Power of Gems and Crystals: How they can transform your life
Soozi Holbeche
The Power of Your Dreams   Soozi Holbeche
**The Right to be Yourself: How to be assertive and make changes in
your life**   Tobe Aleksander

For a free brochure with further information on our range of titles,
please write to:

Piatkus Books
Freepost 7 (WD 4505)
London W1E 4EZ

About the author

Dr Arthur Jackson has a behavioural medicine practice in Sydney, Australia, where he specialises in stress-related illness and teaches self-hypnosis and relaxation techniques. He is past president of the Australian Society of Hypnosis and has published numerous articles on the treatment of anxiety. He conducts workshops and seminars on stress and lectures extensively on this topic all over the world. Among Dr Jackson's patients are international sports stars – including members of the Australian Cricket Team – and executives of major corporations.